COVID: VIRUSES/ VACCINES—

COVID-19 Outbreak Worldwide Pandemic

To order additional copies of this book, contact:
Xlibris
844-714-8691
www.Xlibris.com
Orders@Xlibris.com

ISBN: 978-1-6698-6391-5 (sc)
ISBN: 978-1-6698-6392-2 (hc)
ISBN: 978-1-6698-6390-8 (e)

Library of Congress Control Number: 2023901676

Print information available on the last page

Rev. date: 04/03/2023

My parents for their blessings from the heavens

Our families, students, and colleagues
who inspired us to visualize the need and create
the teaching material for the education of our children

Madan L. Nagpal and Mrs. Raman Nagpal

CONTENTS

PREFACE

As we see that the world goes on, life goes on, and even the tiniest lives survive and are blessed just as do our human lives. The tiny that they are invisible to the human eye makes them difficult to be spotted and studied by the scientists. It was a challenge to see and study COVID-19.

The challenge suggests a range of ideas. The ideas give clues that lead to actions—the paths of life, the roads in the woods of life, and so on.

Here are a few lines from Robert Frost's "The Road Not Taken":

Two roads diverged in a yellow wood,
And sorry I could not travel both
And be one traveler, long I stood
And looked down one as far as I could

Then took the other, as just as fair,
And having perhaps the better claim,
Because it was grassy and wanted wear
Yet knowing how way leads on to way,

I doubted if I should ever come back.
I shall be telling this with a sigh
Somewhere ages and ages hence

And that has made all the difference.

In the book, you will find problems and solutions concerning viruses—outbreaks of viral diseases, working of the immune system, vaccines, drugs to cure, the economic impact of the COVID epidemic, mental health, testing for COVID, pills to treat SARS-CoV-2, the emergence of variants, epidemiological approaches, and much more.

I convey my appreciation to the publisher, Xlibris Corporation, particularly, Yza Garcia, Senior Publishing Consultant, Xlibris.

I hope this book will be incredibly powerful and useful to give a comprehensive account of viruses and the COVID-19 global epidemic.

ACKNOWLEDGMENTS

My wonderful wife Raman Nagpal.
Our amazing son and his charming wife, our daughter-in-law

CHAPTER 1

COVID-19 OUTBREAK

"You must understand the whole life
Not just one little part of it
That is why you must read
That is why you must look at the skies
That is why you must sing and dance
And write poems
And suffer
And understand
For all that is life" Jiddu Krishnamurti

COVID-19 outbreak has become a worldwide pandemic. This book "CO-VI-D: Viruses/Vaccines" provides new and unique approach to the discussion of viruses and vaccines in the recent advent of Corona virus.

COVID-19 disease is a novel viral disease that was first identified in Wuhan, China. The World Health Organization (WHO) announced its official name, Coronavirus disease 2019, abbreviated as COVID-19; 'CO' stands for 'Corona', 'VI' stands for 'Virus', and 'D' stands for 'Disease'. Globally, more than 10 million people are reported to be infected by COVID-19 (WHO Coronavirus Disease Dashboard, 2020).

Centers for Disease Control and Prevention (CDC, USA, 2020) (provided guidelines on how to reduce the risk of infection. It has been discovered that some people get really very sick and die, whereas to some people nothing happens even though they test positive for the virus.

Through this book, we intend to explore etiology, development, and treatment of the COVID-19 disease. The specific topics will give details that could help in understanding symptoms, immunity, worldwide spread and treatments so that we could beat this invisible dangerous beast, the COVID-19.

Adhikari et al. (2020) have given a scoping review of clinical manifestation and diagnosis, prevention and control of COVID-19 during the early outbreak period. The genesis of Corona virus disease happened in December, 2019 when workers in Huanan South China Seafood Market in China suffered with pneumonia, and the Chinese Center for Disease Control and Prevention (China CDC) responded and conducted epidemiological and etiological investigations. The virus was identified and the first genome of COVID-19 was published (Wu F, et al., 2020). It spread like a pandemic similar to Severe Acute Respiratory Syndrome (SARS) and Middle East respiratory syndrome (MERS) coronaviruses.

Coronaviruses (CoVs) belong to family Coronaviridae, and subfamily Orthocoronavirinae. Coronaviruses consist of a group of enveloped, non-segmented, positive-sense single-stranded RNA viruses (Coronaviridae study group of the International Committee on taxonomy of viruses. 2020).

Coronaviruses have RNA as the genetic element that encodes viral proteins involved in transcribing viral RNA, replication, structure, and accessory proteins; spike, envelope, membrane, and nucleocapsids–important for the virus to enter and replicate in the host cell. The accessory proteins are also the main molecules used for diagnosis, antiviral treatment, and potential vaccines (Li F, et al., 2016).

There are three main transmission routes for the COVID-19; droplets transmission, contact transmission, and aerosol transmission. Droplets are expelled through mouth or nose when people talk or breathe. Contact transmission when infected person comes in close contact with another person. Aerosol transmissions occur over long distances and extended time. Most infections are linked to inhalation of droplets containing the virus. The risk of infections is high in crowded and enclosed places. (Carone M, et al., 2021).

The most common symptoms of COVID-19 infection are fever, cough, myalgia or fatigue, pneumonia, and complicated dyspnea, whereas less common reported symptoms include headache, diarrhea, hemoptysis, runny nose, and phlegm producing cough. Patients do recover Diagnostic procedures: Real-time fluorescence (RT-PCR) to detect the positive nucleic acid of SARS-CoV-2 in sputum, throat swabs, and secretions of the lower respiratory tract samples.

The World Health Organization issued detailed guidelines on the use of face masks in the community, during care at home, and in the health care settings of COVID-19. Health care workers are recommended to use particulate respirators such as those certified N95 or FFP2 when performing aerosol-generating procedures and to use medical masks while providing any care to suspected or confirmed cases (Chung et al., 2021).

The evidence so far indicates that COVID-19 is a new viral strain; the alignment of its nucleotide sequences with any other known viruses has not been found and its biological source has not yet been detected. Moreover, COVID-19 has a wide range of symptoms in human ranging from no symptoms to death. Why is it so? Besides age and health of the host person, some genomic scenarios suggest that it has human retroviruses characteristics (HERVs). It is suggested that intensive studies are needed to survey human populations (especially elders and immune compromised, and the link to their predisposition for autoimmune diseases, cancer, and their risk for exogenous viral infection (El-Shehawi AM, et al., 2020). The sequencing of the human genome revealed that at least 1% of the human genome consists of endogenous retroviral sequences, representing past encounters with retroviruses during the course of human evolution. Infectious diseases pose the greatest threat to public health and result in more years of life lost from premature death than any other disease process (World Health Organization, 2004, 2009).

https://www.who.int/healthinfo/global_burden_disease/

GBD_report_2004update_full.pdf

COVID-19 is the ongoing pandemic that has upended our entire planet in unimagined just a few short months (Morens DM & Fauci AS, 2020). Dr. Anthony Stephen Fauci is The chief Medical Advisor to the President, Jo Biden, and the Director of the U.S. National Institute of Allergy and Infectious Diseases (NIAID). President Biden announced June, 2021, as the "Month Of Action" to get USA to 70% of adults vaccinated by Independence Day, July 4, 2021(www.docwirenews.com, June 3, 2021).

Johns Hopkins University-Coronavirus Resource Center (jhu.edu) experts have been at the forefront of the international response to COVID-19. Their project is supported by Bloomberg Philanthropies and the Stavros Niarchos Foundation (SNF). This project is a resource to help advance the understanding of the virus, inform the public, and brief policymakers in order to guide a response, improve care, and save lives. (COVID-19 Resource Center: Expertise and Basic Information. 2021).

The COVID-19 is mutating, as new mutants and variants have been identified. The COVID-19 variants found in the UK, South Africa and Brazil – more properly referred to as the B.1.1.7, B.1.135 and P.1 variants – are examples. All are reported to have significantly higher transmission rates than earlier lineages (Theconversation.com, 2021). A new naming system using Greek alphabets for variants of COVID-19 has been announced by the World Health Organization (WHO). The B.1.1.7 variant is named as "Alpha", the B.1.351 variant is named as "beta", the P.1variant is named as "gamma", and the B.1.617.2 variant is named as "delta" (Newscientist.com, 2021, June1).

COVID-19 risk has been categorized in 4 levels by CDC.gov. Level 1: Lowest level risk, Active exposure and spread; Level 2: High exposure and spread; Level 3: Very high exposure and spread; Level 4: Severe exposure and spread. Households should assume that if one person is sick, every person living there should take appropriate measures to control the spread, which should include self-quarantining and contacting a doctor.

How to overcome COVID-19 Pandemic? CDC.gov has been updating the guidelines on how to protect yourself and others from COVID-19. There are guidelines if you are fully vaccinated, or if not, get vaccinated, and in the meantime, use preventive measures, such as masks, sanitizers, social distancing, etc. Pretty soon we will overcome this pandemic outbreak of the disease. Experts say that the new normal will be far more tech-driven accompanied with sweeping social changes and healthcare reforms (Pewresearch.org, 2021).

References:

Adhikari SP, Meng S, Wu Y, et al. 2020 Epidemiology, causes, clinical manifestation and diagnosis, prevention and control of coronavirus disease (COVID-19) during the early outbreak period: a scoping review. Infect Dis Poverty 9(1):29. doi: 10.1186/s40249-020-00646-x

Carbone M, Lednicky J, Xiao SY et al. 2021 Coronavirus 2019 infectious disease epidemic: Where We Are, What Can Be Done and Hope For. J Thoracic Oncol 16(4):546-571.

CDC, USA, 2020 https://www.cdc.gov/media/releases/2020/t0625-COVID-19-update.html)

Chung JY, Thone MN, Kwon YJ 2021 COVID-19 vaccines: The status and perspectives in delivery points of view. Advanced Drug Delivery Reviews. 170:1-25.

Coronaviridae study group of the International Committee on taxonomy of viruses. 2020 The species Severe Acute Respiratory Syndrome-related coronavirus: classifying 2019-nCoV and naming it SARS-Cov-2. Nat Microbiol 5(4): 536-544.

COVID-19 Resource Center: Expertise and Basic Information. 2021 A collection of COVID-19 content from Health Affairs Journal articles. www.healthaffairs.org.

COVID-19 Resource Center: Expertise and Basic Information. 2021 Johns Hopkins University (jhu.edu).

El-Shehawi AM, Alotaibi SS, Elseehy MM 2020 Genomic study of COVID-19 Corona virus excludes its origin from recombination or characterized biological sources and suggests a role for HERVS in Its wide range symptoms. Cytology and Genetics. 54(6): 588-604. https://doi.org/10.3103/S0095452720060031

Li F. 2016 Structure, function, and evolution of Coronavirus Spike Proteins. Annu Rev Virol 3:237-261. doi: 10.1146/annurev-virology-110615-042301

Morens DM, Fauci AS. 2020 Emerging pandemic diseases: how we got to

COVID-19. Cell 182:1077-1092.

Newscientist.com, 2021, June1. Coronavirus: WHO announces Greek alphabet naming scheme for variants. Pewresearch.org, 2021. Experts-say-the-new-normal-in-2025.

Theconversation.com, 2021(https://theconversation.com/how-the-coronavirus-mutates-and-what-this-means-for-the-future-of-covid-19-154499).

World Health Organization 2004 Global burden of disease. Pages 1-160, 2004 update. www.who.int/healthinfo/global_burden.

World Health Organization 2009 Global health risks: mortality and burden of disease attributable to selected major risks. World Health Organization. https://apps.who.int/iris/handle/10665/44203

Wu, F., Zhao, S., Yu, B., et al. 2020. A new coronavirus associated with human respiratory disease in China.Nature 579 (7798):265-269. https://doi.org/10.1038/s41586-020-2008-3

www.docwirenews.com, June 3, 2021)

CHAPTER 2

OUTBREAKS OF VIRAL DISEASES

The current COVID-19 virus outbreak globally in a very short period is an unprecedented crisis. In order to get hold of it, we need to understand the viruses in general, along with the microbial diseases.

It is not easy to determine whether an infection is microbial or viral as the symptoms could be similar. Diagnosis of microbial (bacterial/fungal) or viral requires other physical tests (body temperature, skin tests, etc.), blood or urine tests and culture tests to identify viruses or bacteria.

Viruses and bacteria have many characteristics in common. They spread by contact with infected people or animals or contaminated things (surfaces, food, water, etc.).

We are going to discuss some of the main outbreaks that caused havoc in the past and millions of people died because of that.

The viral diseases could spread as endemic, pandemic, or epidemic in the world.

Endemic: Endemic is when a limited number of cases occur in a limited area. For example, smallpox occurs as a hemorrhagic form of the disease in children. Smallpox can also become a pandemic as it is a contagious disease.

Epidemic: Epidemic is when the spread of the disease is limited to a region.

Pandemic*:* Pandemic is when a disease outbreak spreads across countries or continents. The World Health Organization (WHO) declared COVID-19 to be a pandemic when it became clear that the illness was severe and that it was spreading quickly over a wide area.

Pandemic (from Lain, pandemus) means pertaining to all people, later came in Greek, meaning all, every, whole, all-inclusive.

The WHO's pandemic alert system ranges from phase 1 (a low risk) to phase 6 (a full pandemic) (webmed.com, 2022):

> **Phase 1:** A virus in animals has caused no known infections in humans.

Phase 2: An animal virus has caused infection in humans.

Phase 3: There are scattered cases or small clusters of disease in humans. If the illness is spreading from human to human, it's not broad enough to cause community-level outbreaks.

Phase 4: The disease is spreading from person to person with confirmed outbreaks at the community level.

Phase 5: The disease is spreading between humans in more than one country of one of the WHO regions.

Phase 6: At least one more country, in a different region from Phase 5, has community-level outbreaks.

Outbreak of viral diseases: Smallpox was the first human viral disease that spread like wildfire. The first smallpox case was recorded in 1977. The World Health Organization (WHO) Global Smallpox Eradication Program resulted in the complete eradication of this disease through the vaccination programs.

The name smallpox is derived from the Latin word for spotted and refers to the raised bumps on the face and body of the patient.

Smallpox is caused by the Variola virus (VARV), a member of the genus *Orthopoxvirus*, in the Poxviridae family.

There are three most common viruses of Poxviridae family:

Smallpox (caused by Viriola virus), **chickenpox** (caused by Varicella virus), and **cowpox** (caused by CPXV).

"The earliest evidence of smallpox comes from ancient Egypt circa 1157 BCE, where the mummified remains of a pockmarked Ramses V were uncovered. International traders spread smallpox throughout the Old World during the 4th-15th centuries CE, while European explorers and conquerors brought the disease to the Western Hemisphere in the early 16th century.

Smallpox directly and profoundly influenced the course of human history. Its tremendous morbidity and mortality led to indiscriminate killing of kings and warlords and tipped the balance of power with regularity in Europe and elsewhere. As a result of smallpox infection, whole civilizations, including the Incas and the Aztecs, were destroyed in a single generation, and efforts to ward off the disease indelibly affected the practice of religion and medicine" (https://emedicine.medscape.com/article/237229-overview, updated on July 28, 2020).

In 1790s, Edward Jenner provided the first exhaustive descriptions of human cowpox in the publication of "An Inquiry Into the Causes and Effects of the Variolae Vaccinae or Cow-Pox" (1798).

Although smallpox and chickenpox share many common characteristics, there are several distinguishing features that help differentiate between the two diseases.

"The general distribution of the fully developed rash of smallpox is *centrifugal*, with more lesions on the arms and legs than on the trunk. The palms and soles are commonly affected.

However, the rash of chickenpox has a *centripetal* distribution, with more lesions on the trunk, with the hands and soles exhibiting few or no lesions.

Moreover, chickenpox is usually mild, whereas smallpox is usually deadly.

U.S.A. government keeps enough smallpox vaccine to protect every person in the United States and recently the drug, TECOVIRIMAT (TPOXX) was approved to treat anyone who may contract the virus" (medscape.com, 2020).

The Dengue virus pandemic: Dengue virus (DENV) belongs to the family Flaviviridae, genus *Flavivirus.* Dengue fever is known for more than 200 years. Worldwide about 50 million cases of dengue infection occur each year, with 22,000 deaths, mostly in children. Dengue fever used to be called break-bone fever because it causes severe joint and muscle pain that feels like bones are breaking (www.niaid.nih.gov/diseases-conditions/dengue-fever,2021). DENV spreads through female mosquitos.

There are three phases of clinical illness of dengue infection: febrile, critical (leakage), and convalescence. The febrile phase is mostly symptomatic. Dengue patients usually have high sustained fever ranging from two to seven days, mean duration of four to five days. Common signs and symptoms are severe headache, retro-orbital pain, body ache (myalgia), arthralgia/joint pain, and minor bleeding manifestations, such as petechiae, epistaxis, gum bleeding, and coffee-ground vomiting.

The Spanish influenza pandemic: The Spanish influenza pandemic of 1918–1919 caused around 50 million deaths worldwide. It spread through United Kingdom, France, Spain, and Italy during the end of World War I. In addition, its socioeconomic consequences were huge. This was probably caused by a mutated strain of the virus, which was carried from the port city of Plymouth in south-western England by ships. Deadly clusters of symptoms were recorded, including nasal hemorrhage, pneumonia, and encephalitis.

Discovery of virus: In 1918, a virus was defined scientifically to be a submicroscopic infectious entity which could be filtered but not grown *in vitro*. In the 1880s Pasteur developed an attenuated vaccine for the rabies virus by serial passageway ahead of his time. Ivanoski's works on the tobacco mosaic virus in 1890s led to the discovery of the virus. He found an infectious agent that acted as a microorganism as it multiplied yet passed through the sterilizing filter as a non-microbe. By the 1910s several viruses, defined as filterable infectious microbes, had been identified as causing infectious disease.

.The HIV/AIDS pandemic: The HIV/AIDS Pandemic claimed more than 39 million lives worldwide as on June 07, 2021. Human immunodeficiency viruses (HIVs) cause Auto Immune Deficiency Syndrome (AIDS). HIVs are of two types, HIV-1 group and HIV-2 group. Both HIVs originated as a result of multiple cross-species transmissions of simian immune deficiency viruses (SIVs) naturally infecting African primates.

HIVs weaken a person's ability to fight infections. HIVs are mostly contracted through unprotected sex or needle sharing ("AIDS and HIV Center," *WebMD*, 2022).

Antiretroviral therapy (ART) has substantially reduced HIV-related morbidity and mortality, improved long-term outcomes for people with HIV and plays a key role in HIV prevention.

The Ebola virus pandemic: The Ebola virus was first discovered in 1976 near the Ebola River in Congo. Since then, the virus has been infecting people from time to time. Ebola virus disease (EVD) is a deadly disease with occasional outbreaks. It is caused by a group of viruses within the Genus Ebolavirus (species: Zaire Ebola virus, Bombali Ebola virus).

"An epidemic of the Zaire species of Ebola virus emerged in West Africa in 2014 and lasted for 2 years. It was one of the worst world's deadliest epidemics, resulting in 29,000 cases and 11,000 fatalities" (https://www.who.int, cited 2022).

The Zika virus pandemic: "Zika virus (ZIKV) caused widespread epidemic in 2015 in Central America. Zika virus (ZIKV) is a flavivirus (Flaviviridae family) transmitted by mosquitos. Its name was derived from the Zika Forest in Uganda where it was isolated in 1947 from the serum of a Rhesus monkey. The ZIKV caused microcephaly in fetuses born to mothers infected with it" (www.nih.gov., 2016).

"The recent rapid spread of Zika virus and its unexpected linkage to birth defects and an autoimmune-neurological syndrome has generated worldwide concern. Zika virus is a flavivirus like dengue, yellow fever and West Nile viruses. The structure of Zika virus is similar to other known flavivirus structures except for the ~10 amino acids that surround the Asn154 glycosylation site found in each of the 180 envelope glycoproteins that make up the icosahedral shell. The carbohydrate moiety associated with this residue, recognizable in the cryo-EM electron density, may function as an attachment site of the virus to host cells" (Source).

The COVID-19 pandemic: COVID-19 is a novel Coronavirus pandemic that has infected globally more than 100 million people and killed 2 million people as of April 2021.

The COVID-19 infection "starts with the basic flu symptoms, but it could eventually affect your lungs, liver, kidneys, and even your brain" (www. webmd.com, 2021).

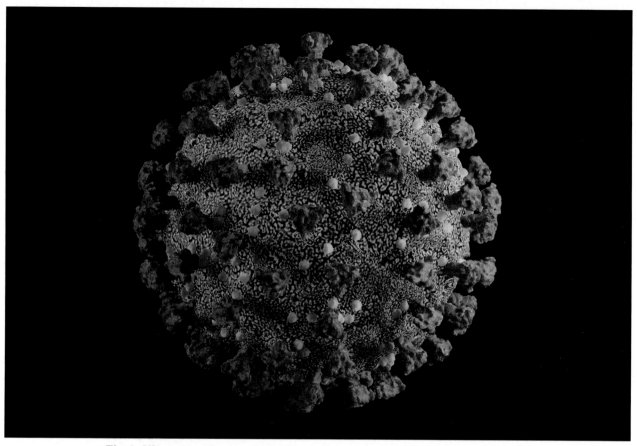

Fig.1: Ultrastructural morphology of Coronavirus (Public Health Image Library: https://phil.cdc.gov/Details.aspx?pid=23311, 2020).

Coronavirus as viewed under the electron microscope has spikes on the outer surface of the virus. It is a novel virus named severe acute respiratory syndrome coronavirus 2 (SARS-CoV-2) It was identified as the cause of the outbreak of respiratory illness first detected in Wuhan, China, in 2019.

COVID-19 is the disease caused by the novel coronavirus—SARS-Cov-2— that results in a variety of symptoms, such as fever, cough, and a list of physical and mental problems. Some people develop mild or no symptoms while others get seriously ill.

The typical symptoms of COVID-19 disease:

The typical symptoms are fever, shortness of breath, loss of smell or taste, body aches and pains, headache, sore throat, runny or stuffy nose, as well as digestive symptoms, such as nausea, vomiting, or diarrhea

Infected individuals are highly contagious and can transmit the disease even if they are asymptomatic.

The Centers for Disease Control and Prevention (CDC) in the USA and the World Health Organization (WHO) currently advise the public to call their doctor if they believe they have been exposed to COVID-19 or exhibit fever and cough.

Treatment of COVID-19 disease:

The National Institutes of Health (NIH) published COVID-19 treatment guidelines. For treatment, there are three categories:

Mild illness. Fever and cough, but no shortness of breath and difficulty in breathing.

Moderate illness. The individual also has a lower respiratory illness, such as pneumonia.

Severe illness. The individual also has low blood oxygen levels that are less than 94 percent, a higher breathing rate, and signs of severe lung infection

According to CDC, 81 percent of people with mild or moderate illness recover at home. On the other hand, if not taken care of, the symptoms may worsen leading to more serious illness.

Asymptomatic infections. It is estimated that about 20 percent of COVID-19 infections are asymptomatic but still contagious. It is critical to continue practicing good hygiene, physical distancing, and mask-wearing to reduce the spread of the virus.

Who should get tested? Anyone who has any symptoms of COVID-19 should get tested even if the symptoms are very mild. Other situations where testing is recommended include

Close contact. It's important to get tested if you have been in close contact with someone that has confirmed COVID-19. This means you've been within 6 feet of them for fifteen minutes or longer over a twenty-four-hour period.

High-risk activities. Some activities can put you at a higher risk of contracting SARS-CoV-2 and becoming ill with COVID-19, so it is important to get tested after doing things like traveling or attending a large gathering.

Testing referral. It is possible that your healthcare provider may ask you to get tested, such as prior to a surgery or procedure (CDC.gov, 2021).

Getting Tested for COVID-19. CDC has an update on the diagnostic procedures for COVID-19 infections (CDC.gov, 2021, updated on May 4, 2021).

Viral test checks specimens are withdrawn from the individual's nose or mouth and viral tests are performed in a laboratory, at a testing site or at home or anywhere else.

Two types of viral tests are used

1. Antigen tests

2. Nucleic acid amplification tests (NAATs)

Signs that you need medical attention. COVID-19 can progress into a serious illness in some people. Some of the warning signs of serious illness to look out for include difficulty in breathing, pain or pressure in the chest, or other signs of COVID-19 infection. If you or someone else develops these symptoms, call 911 or your local emergency services immediately. Be sure to let the emergency dispatcher know that you're seeking medical attention for someone that has or may have COVID-19

The highly transmissible Delta variant is now the dominant strain of COVID-19 in the United States (Centers for Disease Control and Prevention, 2021, CDC 24/7, Save lives, Protecting People). As of July 3, 2021, the Delta variant accounted for 51.7 percent of new COVID-19 cases that had been genetically sequenced. Tw o weeks earlier, on June 19, 2021, the Delta variant accounted for 30 percent of new cases.

COVID-19 vaccines have been developed by a number of companies and are found very effective against Delta variants and other variants of COVID-19. I hope it will end the COVID-19 pandemic in the USA and around the world.

CHAPTER 3

FUNDAMENTALS OF VIRUSES

Here we will discuss the basic elements and the common features of the viruses that constitute the fundamentals of viruses. We will identify and classify the viruses on the basis of their features. We have to learn the fundamentals of the structure and function of different viruses that could lead us to their usefulness to us. We could then control and manipulate the viruses to our advantage.

Here are the common features of viruses that we are going to discuss in this chapter:

1. the sizes of the viruses

2. the invasion of viruses of the host cells

1. The sizes of the viruses

Viruses are small and range over many magnitudes. A virus is smaller than a bacterium or a human cell. Most viruses range in size from 5 to 300 nanometers (nm). For example,

Picornaviruses (ssRNA naked) range in size from 20 to 30 nm,

Coronaviruses (ssRNA enveloped) are 80 to 160 nm;

Herpesviruses (dsDNA enveloped) are 150 to 200 nm.

Many giant viruses are known as well. For example, Mimivirus, *Acanthamoeba polyphaga Mimivirus*, is the largest known virus. It is 750 nm in diameter and has dsDNA with a genome of ~1.2 Mbp.

After the discovery of Mimivirus, further sampling of various environments and geographical locations led to the isolation of Moumouvirus chilensis and Megavirus chilensis ~500 nm, 1.26 Mb, with a full transcription apparatus allowing them to replicate in the host's cytoplasm. Pandoraviruses have genomes of up to 2.8 Mb and sizes of ~1000 nm.

Another giant virus, named *Pithovirus sibericum*, was isolated from a >30,000-y-old radiocarbon-dated sample of the virome of Siberian permafrost. The revival of such an ancestral amoeba-infecting virus used as a safe indicator of the possible presence of pathogenic DNA viruses, suggests that the thawing of permafrost either from global warming or industrial exploitation of circumpolar regions might not be exempt from future threats to human or animal health. For thousands of years, viruses remained entirely frozen. Viruses, by definition, are not alive but are inert particles. Until 2003, it was thought that all viruses were tiny and completely invisible under a standard light microscope. Since then, several giant viruses have been discovered, including Moumouviruses, Pandoraviruses, and Pithoviruses. Pithoviruses are astonishing 1.5 micrometers long. Pithovirus is easily visible under a microscope as an oval rimmed by a dark black envelope with a perforated plug at the end, about the size of a bacterial cell. The virus enters the amoebae cells, hijacks the cells' metabolic machinery to create many copies of it, and splits the cells open, killing them and freeing itself to infect further cells. The researchers say that it indicates that giant viruses are much more common and more diverse than was previously thought.

Another fundamental feature of viruses is that they invade the cells.

2. The invasion of viruses of the host cells

Viruses invade living cells. Viruses begin a new cycle of infection by a number of ways depending upon the virus and the host. Viruses initially stick to cell membranes through interactions. The virus surfs along the fluid surface of the cell and eventually the viral fusion proteins bind to receptor molecules on the cell membrane.

We will discuss a few significantly important viruses that play vital roles in our lives.

How does the influenza virus invade a host cell? The entry of influenza viruses includes a number of steps in host cell infection. Hemagglutinin (HA) is a trimeric glycoprotein that is present in multiple copies in the membrane envelope of influenza virus. HA contains a fusion peptide, a receptor binding site, a metastable structural motif, and the transmembrane domain. The first step of influenza virus entry is the recognition of the host cell receptor molecule, terminal α-sialic acid, by HA. This multivalent attachment by multiple copies of trimetric HA triggers endocytosis of influenza virus that is contained in the endosome. The endosome-trapped virus traffics via a unidirectional pathway to near the nucleus. At this location, the interior pH of the endosome becomes acidic that induces a dramatic conformational change in HA to insert the fusion peptide into the host membrane, induce juxtaposition of the two membranes, and form a fusion pore that allows the release of the genome segments of influenza virus. HA plays a key role in the entire entry pathway.

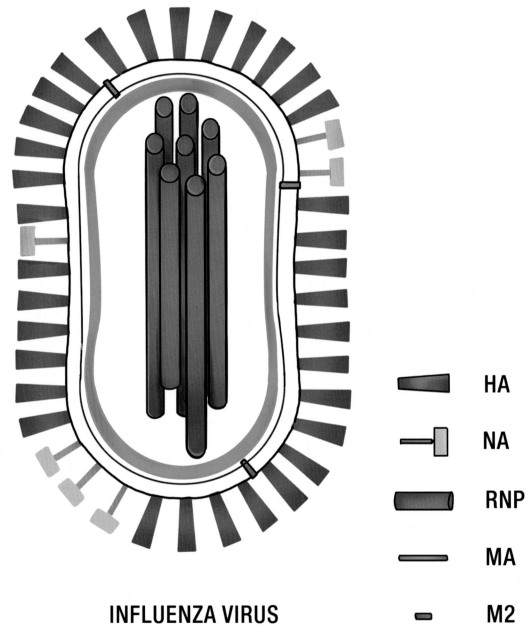

HA

NA

RNP

MA

INFLUENZA VIRUS

M2

Fig.2: Cartoon showing the architecture of influenza virus (Luo M, 2012).

How do coronaviruses (CoVs) invade cells? The primary determinants of CoVs tropism are the S protein, which binds to the membrane receptors, such as Angiotensin-converting enzyme 2 (ACE2), CD147, also known as Basigin or EMMPRIN, a transmembrane glycoprotein on the host cells.

Large conformational changes in the S-protein result in S1 shedding and exposure of the fusion machinery in S2. Class I fusion proteins, such as the CoV-2 S-protein, undergo large conformational changes during the fusion process and must, by necessity, be highly flexible and dynamic. Indeed, cryo-EM structures of the SARS-CoV-2 spike reveal considerable flexibility and dynamics in the S1 subunit, especially around the RBD.

The invasion of HIV viruses of the host cells: In 1981, AIDS was diagnosed, and 3 years later, Luc Montagnier of the Pasteur Institute of Paris and Robert Gallo then of the National Cancer Institute discovered that the infection by HIV virus caused AIDS.

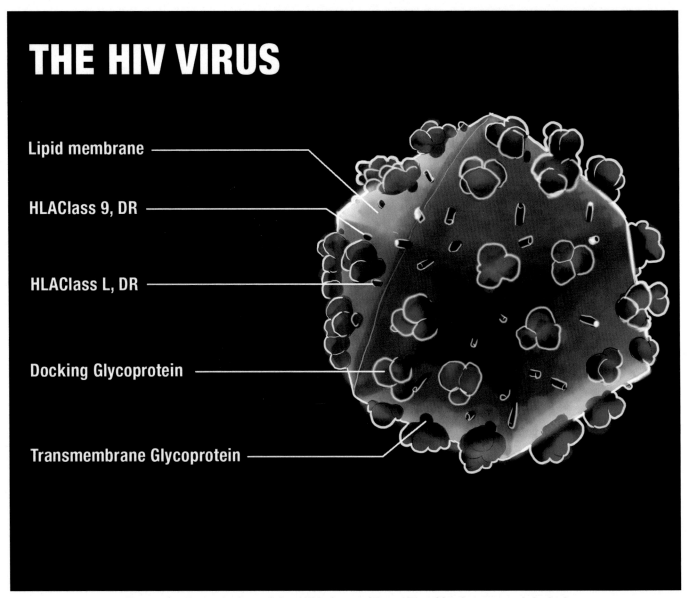

THE HIV VIRUS

Lipid membrane

HLAClass 9, DR

HLAClass L, DR

Docking Glycoprotein

Transmembrane Glycoprotein

Fig. 3. A 3D rendering of the HIV virus with some of its key parts labeled (Image credit: www.3Dscience.com, searched on February 6, 2022).

The French virologist Luc Montagnier and joint recipient H. Hausen received Nobel Prize in Physiology and Medicine in 2008 for his discovery of the human immunodeficiency virus HIV. During the COVID-19 pandemic, Montagnier promoted that SARS-CoV-2 is the causative virus.

The invasion of herpes viruses of the host cells. Herpesviruses (Herpesviridae) is a large family of dsDNA viruses, which comprise 8 human pathogens and many additional viruses infecting other species.

"New research revealed how Herpes Simplex Viruses (HSV-1 and HSV-2) invade cells and take control of the cell's machinery to replicate itself and hide from the immune system" (*VCU News,* Virginia Commonwealth University, 2008). HSV-1 usually causes blisters around the mouth and lips, whereas HSV-2 usually causes blisters around the genitals and rectum.

The invasion of hepatitis viruses of the host cells. Hepatitis A virus (HAV) causes a highly contagious liver infection. It spreads from contaminated food or water or contact with someone who is infected.

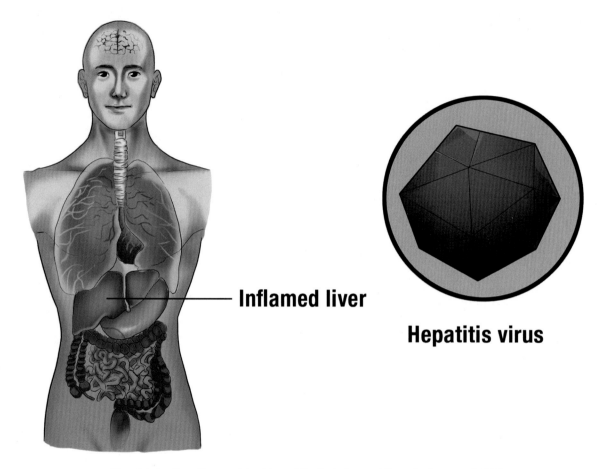

Fig. 4 Infection Caused by Hepatitis A: Inflamed liver (cdc.gov, 2020)

Hepatitis A is preventable by vaccine. Symptoms include inflamed liver, jaundice, fatigue, nausea, abdominal pain, loss of appetite, and low-grade fever. The condition clears up on its own in one or two months. Rest and adequate hydration can help. HAV is found in the stool and blood of people who are infected. "Most people with hepatitis A do not have long-lasting illness. The best way to prevent hepatitis A is to get vaccinated" (cdc.gov., USA, 2020).

Hepatitis viruses are assigned to diverse virus families and genera. Namely, they belong to the families *Picornaviridae*, genus *Hepatovirus* (HAV),

"In general, human and non-human hepatitis virus homologues resemble each other in major genomic properties such as structure of the genomic nucleic acid, open reading frame (ORF) composition, genome length and presence and type of noncoding regions" (Source).

There are 5 kinds of hepatitis viruses (HAV); A, B, C, D, and E, all target the liver but do so in different ways with different outcomes. The reason they all are called hepatitis is because the word itself, from the Greek hepar + it is, means liver inflammation (CDC.gov., USA, 2021).

CHAPTER 4

FUNDAMENTALS OF IMMUNE SYSTEM

The immune system consists of a network of biological processes that protect an organism from diseases, pathogens, viruses, and other foreign cells. The immune system is capable of distinguishing the cells and tissues of other organisms from the host's own healthy tissues and cells. Elie Metchnikoff postulated the concept of self and non-self, referring to what belongs to the body and what does not, and won the Nobel Prize in 1908 in Medicine.

In 1966, it was discovered that T cell-deficient mice failed to reject normal and malignant human tissue. These T cell-deficient mice were hairless nude (nu/nu) mice. In 1968, it was shown that nu/nu mice lacked thymus and thus were devoid of functional T cells. A subsequent series of investigations revealed that the nu/nu phenotype arose from a mutation of the *Foxn1* gene previously known as the *whn* gene (winged-helix nude or Hfh11^{nu}). T cells are critical to the adaptive immune system, where the body adapts specifically to foreign invaders.

The humanized mouse models are being developed for the production of vaccines and therapies to combat viral diseases and other medical problems.

The immune system is made up of a large network of the lymphatic system.

Lymphatic system: "The lymphatic system is a network of delicate tubes throughout the body. It consists of lymph, lymphatic vessels, lymph nodes, lymphatic or lymphoid organs, and lymphoid tissues. The vessels carry a clear fluid called lymph (the Latin word lympha refers to the deity of fresh water, 'Lympha') towards the heart." The lymph is a filtrate formed in the tissues that the network delivers to the central circulation.

The main roles of the lymphatic system are to manage the fluid levels in the body, react to bacteria, deal with cancer cells, deal with cell products that otherwise would result in disease or disorders, absorb some of the fats in our diet from the intestine.

The lymphatic system is made up of lymph nodes (also called lymph glands) -- which trap microbes, lymph vessels -- tubes that carry lymph, the colorless fluid that bathes your body's tissues and contains infection-fighting white blood cells, white blood cells (lymphocytes).

The immune system stockpiles a huge arsenal of cells, not only lymphocytes but also cell-devouring phagocytes. The immune system stores just a few of each kind of the different cells needed to recognize millions of possible enemies. When an antigen appears, those few matching cells multiply into a full-scale army. After their job is done, they fade away, leaving sentries behind to watch for future attacks.

Immune system is associated with the nervous system forming an integrated dynamic network: Immune system is a highly integrated life system, just like nervous system, as they evolve during embryonic development. Both systems, the immune system and nervous system, are regarded as supersystems because they engender themselves by generation from a single progenitor, creating a dynamic self-regulating system. The immune system can make self-nonself discrimination that enables the body to protect itself from microbial organisms in the environment. However, the immune system has become a quite dangerous and harmful life system, providing ample opportunity for errors and undesirable results, e.g. autoimmunity and allergy.

Immune response by the immune system:

The immune system is a dynamic mesh of molecules, cells and tissues spanning the entire organism. The immune system evolved to cope with pathogens anywhere in the body, may it be a parasite residing the gut or a virus spreading to multiple organs.

Antigens: The immune system protects the body from possibly harmful substances by recognizing and responding to the antigens. Antigens are substances (usually proteins) on the surface of cells, viruses, fungi, or bacteria. Antigens are the pathogens. These could be nonliving substances such as chemicals, drugs, and foreign particles (such as a splinter). The immune system recognizes and destroys, or tries to destroy, substances that contain antigens.

Our body's cells have proteins that are antigens. These include a group of antigens called human leucocyte antigens (HLA). These are coded by the short arm of chromosome 6. The differences in HLA between the donor and recipient are the primary causes for rejection of transplant. HLA class I is present on the surface of all nucleated cells, whereas HLA class II is present on specialized Antigen-presenting Cells (APC). The HLA is also known as the human version of the major histocompatibility complex (MHC) found in all higher vertebrates.

Immune Defense Systems: There are four distinct aspects of the immune response, innate, adaptive, acquired, and passive. All work together to protect against pathogens.

Innate Immunity: Innate immunity is the body's first reaction to an invader. It is known to be a nonspecific and quick response to any sort of pathogen. Innate immunity involves barriers that keep harmful materials from entering your body. These barriers form the first line of defense in the immune response.

Components of the innate immune response include physical barriers like the skin and mucous membranes, immune cells such as neutrophils, macrophages, and monocytes, and soluble factors including cytokines, interferons, and complements. The soluble forms make up the innate humoral immunity.

Adaptive Immunity: The adaptive immunity is specific as its response caters to antigens and thus, it takes longer to activate the components involved.

Acquired Immunity: Acquired immunity is immunity that develops with exposure to various antigens. The immune system builds a defense against that specific antigen.

Passive immunity: Passive immunity develops when an individual receives antiserum from another source. An infant develops passive immunity because it gets antiserum through the placenta from its mother. Several products have been approved by the U.S. Food and Drug Administration (FDA) for passive immunization and immunotherapy, including antibodies against botulism, diphtheria, hepatitis A, hepatitis B, measles, rabies, Kawasaki disease, and tetanus (CDC.gov., USA, 2021).

Components of Immune System: The immune system includes certain types of white blood cells, also called lymphocytes. The immune system also includes chemicals and proteins in the blood, such as antibodies, complement proteins, and interferons. Some of these directly attack foreign substances in the body, and others work together to help the immune system cells.

Components of the adaptive immunity include cells such as dendritic cells, T cells, B cells, as well as antibodies also known as immunoglobulins, which directly interact with antigens and are a very important component for a strong response against an invader.

Lymphocytes are of two types, B lymphocytes and T lymphocytes.

B lymphocytes produce antibodies.

Antibodies: Antibodies help the body to fight microbes or the toxins (poisons) they produce. They do this by recognizing substances called antigens on the surface of the microbe, or in the chemicals they produce, which mark the microbe or toxin as being foreign. Antibodies attach to a specific antigen and make it easier for the immune cells to destroy the antigen. There are many cells, proteins and chemicals involved in this attack.

T lymphocytes attack antigens directly and help control the immune response. They also release chemicals, known as cytokines, which control the entire immune response.

Natural Killer (NK) cells: NK cells are a part of the innate immune response to viral infections. NK cells are best characterized by their cytotoxic function and their ability to produce cytokines upon stimulation. With respect to their cytotoxic potential, they target infected, transformed, and stressed cells. In this way, they not only eliminate unwanted cells but also contribute to cellular homeostasis. The conventional known anatomical site of NK cell production is the bone marrow, where interactions with other cellular components, cytokines and soluble molecules support and drive NK cell development. NK cells are early responders to acute SARS-CoV-2 infection, with recruitment of CD56[bright] and CD56[dim] NK cells from the circulation to the lungs.

Innate Lymphoid Cells (ILCs): ILCs are newly identified members of the lymphoid lineage with emerging roles in mediating immune responses and in regulating tissue homeostasis and inflammation.

ILC1s are associated with T helper (Th1), ILC2s are associated with Th2, and ILC3s are associated with Th17 functions.

The group 1 ILC lineage comprises ILCs such as natural killer (NK) cells that produce type 1 cytokines, notably interferon-γ and tumor necrosis factor. The other group 1 ILCs have been reported, mainly *in vitro*, and their physiological roles remain to be defined.

The group 2 ILC population comprises ILC2s, which express interleukin-5 (IL-5) and IL-13 and require GATA-binding protein 3 (GATA3) and retinoic acid receptor-related orphan receptor-α (RORα) for their development. They have crucial roles in protective type 2 immunity to helminth infection. Furthermore, although T helper 2 cells are a major source of type 2 cytokines during allergic asthma, ILC2s also contribute to disease pathology.

ILC3s were first defined as intestinal lymphoid cells that express the NK cell activating receptor NKp46, but otherwise bear little functional resemblance to conventional NK cells, and require RORγ for their development. They express IL-17A and IL-22.

Recent studies have also implicated ILC3s in the development of inflammatory bowel disease. Studies in *Rag2*$^{-/-}$ mice demonstrated that, in the early phase of *Citrobacter rodentium* infection, IL-22 is produced from an innate cell source.

Lymphoid tissue-inducer (LTi) cells are an ILC subset that appears to be closely related to ILC3s, but their exact relationship remains controversial. Together, LTi cells and ILC3s have been classified as group 3 ILCs.

Organs of the Immune System: The biological processes of the immune system are carried out by the various organs of the body. The organs of the immune system are called lymphoid organs, and these are positioned throughout the body. These are the lungs, liver, bone marrow, heart, spleen, thymus, lymph nodes, tonsils, mucous membranes, and skin.

Lungs: Lungs are the key targets for viral infections. The bronchial and alveolar cells of the lungs are constantly exposed to air pathogens. Infected cells produce an immune response in multiple cell types.

The lungs are an important site of host defense immune system. The capillary blood contains an increased concentration of neutrophils and other leukocytes compared with large vessels, due to the structure of the pulmonary capillary bed, the diameter of spherical leukocytes, and their poor deformability compared with erythrocytes. During inflammation within the distal airways, neutrophils sequester within the pulmonary capillaries and emigrate into the parenchyma. This sequential process involves complex events regulating interactions between mechanical and adhesive properties of both neutrophils and endothelial cells. Initial changes in the cytoskeleton may stiffen the neutrophils and prevent them from deforming, while subsequent dynamic cytoskeletal remodeling of neutrophils and endothelial cells results in crawling and transendothelial migration. Emigration of neutrophils can occur through at least two adhesion pathways: one that requires the CD11/CD18 adhesion complex and one that does not. Which pathway is selected is determined by the stimulus and the signaling pathways that are initiated. Migration through the alveolocapillary wall is also highly regulated. Neutrophils released from the bone marrow traffic first through the pulmonary microvasculature, and the phenotype of these newly released neutrophils impacts pulmonary host defense.

These various immune cells can then emigrate to the airway vessels and the capillaries of the virus-infected airway and alveolar compartments. Virus-infected epithelial cells release viral fragments and live viral particles, which are taken up by dendritic cells. These dendritic cells enter the lymphatic vessels and lymph nodes.

The respiratory tract (nose, throat, larynx, trachea, bronchi, and lungs) has a large surface area that is in direct contact with the outside environment. It comprises distinct epithelial cell layers and vascular beds, including the alveolar gas-exchange surfaces of the lung, which contain the largest vascular bed in the body. Different immune cells are recruited to various compartments of virus-infected tissues.

Liver: The liver is the largest solid organ of the human body, accounting for almost 2% of adult body weight and weighing approximately 1.5 kg; it performs an amazing number of tasks that support the function of other organs and impacts all physiologic systems. An essential function of the liver is protein synthesis and metabolism, including the metabolism of amino acids, carbohydrates, lipids and vitamins. However, the liver is also responsible for the removal of pathogens and exogenous antigens from the systemic circulation. The liver protects from antigenic overload of dietary components. The liver is also instrumental to fetal immune tolerance. Loss of liver tolerance leads to the induction of autoimmune liver diseases. Liver-related lymphoid subpopulations also act as critical antigen-presenting cells.

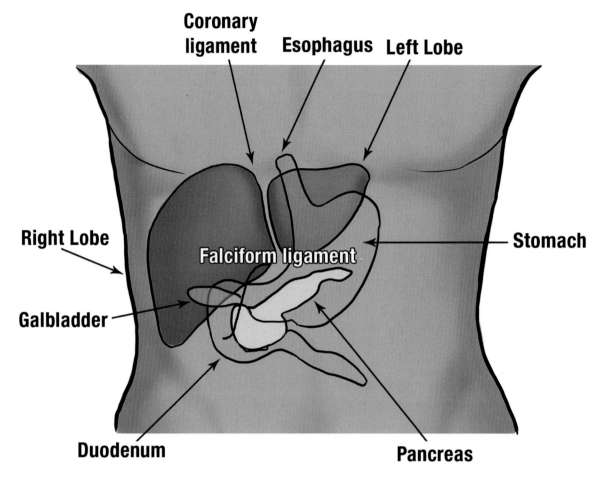

Coronary ligament

Esophagus

Left Lobe

Right Lobe

Falciform ligament

Stomach

Galbladder

Duodenum

Pancreas

Fig 1. Anatomical location and external appearance of the liver (https://www.ncbi.nlm.nih.gov/, 2021)

Bone Marrow: Bone marrow is the soft tissue in the bones. Bone marrow is the primary organ for B cell maturation. Most B cell development takes place in the bone marrow followed by mature cell development in secondary lymphoid organs (SLO) and then eventually circulation in the blood. In the bone marrow, B cells are derived from hematopoietic stem cells and differentiate into lymphoid progenitors.

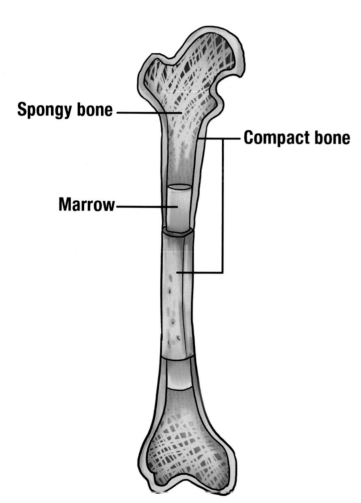

Spongy bone ——

Compact bone

Marrow——

Fig 2. Bone marrow (https://i.pinimg.com/originals/0f/f7/35/0ff73547cf2afff82f5789ab115ca57b.jpg).

Heart: The heart and the circulatory (or cardiovascular) system is a closed network of organs and vessels that moves blood around the body. The primary purposes of the circulatory system are to deliver nutrients, immune factors, and oxygen to tissues and to carry away waste products for elimination.

Under normal circumstances, the circulatory system and the blood should be sterile; the circulatory system has no normal microbiota. Because the system is closed, there are no easy portals of entry into the circulatory system for microbes. Those that are able to breach the body's physical barriers and enter the bloodstream encounter a host of circulating immune defenses, such as antibodies, complement proteins, phagocytes, and other immune cells. Microbes often gain access to the circulatory system through a break in the skin (e.g., wounds, needles, intravenous catheters, insect bites) or spread to the circulatory system from infections in other body sites. For example, microorganisms causing pneumonia or renal infection may enter the local circulation of the lung or kidney and spread from there throughout the circulatory network.

If microbes in the bloodstream are not quickly eliminated, they can spread rapidly throughout the body, leading to serious, even life-threatening infections. The presence of viruses in the blood is called viremia. Microbial toxins can also be spread through the circulatory system, causing a condition termed toxemia.

Microbes and microbial toxins in the blood can trigger an inflammatory response so severe that the inflammation damages host tissues and organs more than the infection itself. This counterproductive immune response is called systemic inflammatory response syndrome (SIRS), and it can lead to the life-threatening condition known as sepsis. Sepsis is characterized by the production of excess cytokines that leads to classic signs of inflammation such as fever, vasodilation, and edema. Certain infections can cause inflammation in the heart and blood vessels. Inflammation of the endocardium, the inner lining of the heart, is called endocarditis and can result in damage to the heart valves severe enough to require surgical replacement. Inflammation of the pericardium, the sac surrounding the heart, is called pericarditis. The term myocarditis refers to the inflammation of the heart's muscle tissue. Pericarditis and myocarditis can cause fluid to accumulate around the heart, resulting in congestive heart failure. Inflammation of blood vessels is called vasculitis. Although somewhat rare, vasculitis can cause blood vessels to become damaged and rupture; as blood is released, small red or purple spots called petechiae appear on the skin. If the damage of tissues or blood vessels is severe, it can result in reduced blood flow to the surrounding tissues. This condition is called ischemia, and it can be very serious. In severe cases, the affected tissues can die and become necrotic; these situations may require surgical debridement or amputation.

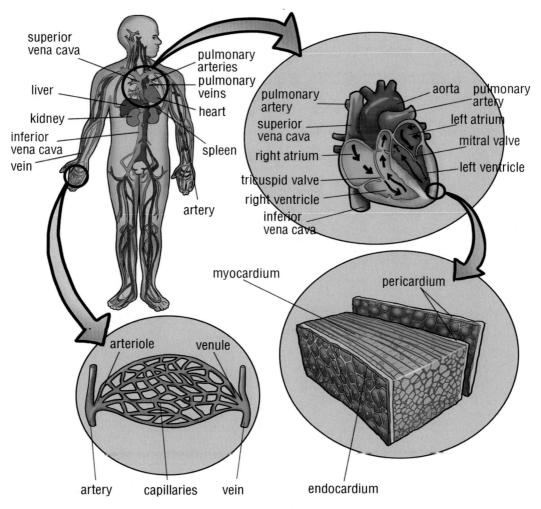

Fig. 3. Heart, the major components of the human circulatory system include the heart, arteries, veins, and capillaries.

Autoimmune heart diseases result when the body's own immune defense system mistakes cardiac antigens as foreign, and attacks them, leading to inflammation of the heart as a whole, or in parts. The most common form of autoimmune heart disease is rheumatic heart disease, or rheumatic fever.

Spleen: The spleen is an organ that filters the blood and is responsible for generating blood-borne immune responses. Spleen is a flattened organ at the upper left of the abdomen. The spleen contains specialized compartments where immune cells gather and work, and serves as a meeting ground where immune defenses confront antigens. The spleen stores various immune system cells. When needed, they move through the blood to other organs. Scavenger cells (phagocytes) in the spleen act as a filter for germs that get into the bloodstream. There is always a lot of blood flowing through the spleen tissue. At the same time this tissue is very soft. In the event of severe injury, for example in an accident, the spleen may rupture easily. Surgery is then usually necessary because otherwise there is a danger of bleeding to death. If the spleen needs to be removed completely, other immune system organs can carry out its roles.

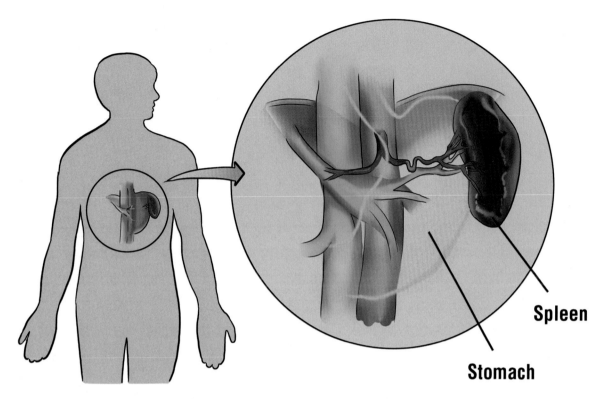

Spleen (https://www.bing.com/images/)
Fig. 4. Spleen, located at the upper left of the abdomen. (https://www.webmd.com/, June 23, 2021).

Thymus: Thymus is a primary lymphoid organ, able to generate mature T cells that eventually colonize secondary lymphoid organs, and is therefore essential for peripheral T cell renewal.

Thymus gland is a small organ situated in the neck of vertebrates that produces T cells for the immune system.

Thymus produces special types of immune system cells, called thymus cell lymphocytes (T cells) that mature in the thymus. Among other tasks, these cells coordinate the processes of the innate and adaptive immune systems. T cells move through the body and constantly monitor the surfaces of all cells for changes. Thymus receives precursor T cells from bone marrow and helps them to mature into full-fledged T cells (such as CD4 and CD8 cells) that are trained to attack foreign cells or pathogens. Thymus gland reaches full maturity only in children, and then it becomes much smaller at the approach of puberty. T cells development and export can be altered as a result of an infectious disease. One common feature is the severe atrophy of the infected organ, mainly due to the apoptosis-related depletion of immature $CD4^+CD8^+$ T cells. A variety of infectious agents; including viruses, protozoa, and fungi, invade the thymus, raising the hypothesis of the generation of central immunological tolerance for at least some of the infectious agent-derived antigens. It seems clear that the thymus is targeted in a variety of infections, and that such targeting may have consequences on the behavior of peripheral T lymphocytes.

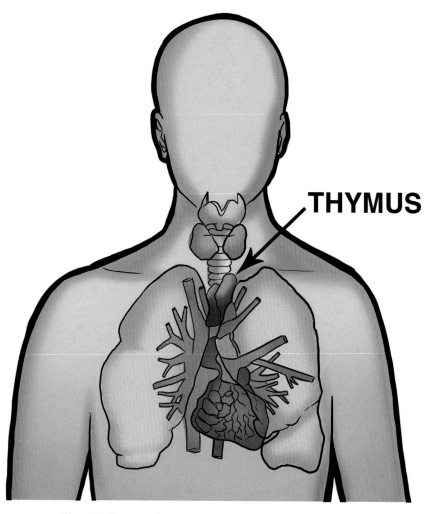

Fig. 5. Thymus (eurostemcell.org, June 2, 2018).

Thymus is close to the heart and larger in babies than in adults. The famous Greek philosopher-surgeon, Galen, noticed that thymus gland changes with age. He found that it is large in newborn babies and becomes smaller when they become adults. It starts to shrink slowly with age, and at the age of seventy-five years, it just disappears.

Surgeons may remove the thymus gland, a thymectomy, under certain conditions. One reason is that a baby is born with a heart problem. The thymus is near the heart and large in babies. So surgeons have to remove it to operate on a baby's heart

Lymph nodes: Lymph nodes are small bean-shaped tissues found along the lymphatic vessels. Lymph nodes contain immune cells that kill foreign invaders, such as viruses. They're an important part of the body's immune system. Lymph nodes are found in various parts of the body, including the neck, armpits, and groin.

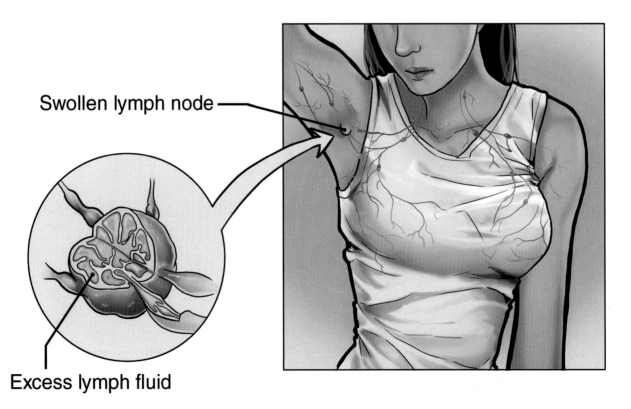

Swollen lymph node

Excess lymph fluid

Fig 6. Swollen lymph node in the armpit (Cleveland Clinic, 2018).

"Swollen lymph node is a sign that your immune system is fighting an infection or illness. Swollen lymph nodes can occur in the armpits, chest, neck, and groin. The most common cause of lymph node swelling in the neck is an upper respiratory infection. The bacteria and viruses that cause Cold and Flu, Sinus infections, Strep throat, Skin wounds, or Mononucleosis, could result in swollen lymph nodes. Swollen lymph node is a symptom and diagnosing it could pinpoint what is causing it. Most of the time the lymph node cells will fight off the virus or bacterium, and gradually the lymph node will shrink back to normal size. In some cases, swollen lymph nodes can even point to cancer (lymphoma) or autoimmune diseases (like lupus, rheumatoid arthritis), sexually transmitted infections (HIV, syphilis), bacterial infections (like lyme disease, typhoid fever), viral infections (measles, Epstein-Barr) or cancer (lymphoma, leukemia). These conditions could require more aggressive treatments over a longer period of time. The swollen lymph nodes may not return to their normal size until after your treatment has ended" (https://my.clevelandclinic.org, 2018).

Tonsils: The tonsils are also part of the immune system. They are located at the throat and palate. They can stop germs entering the body through the mouth or the nose. The tonsils also contain a lot of white blood cells, which are responsible for killing germs. There are different types of tonsils: palatine, adenoid and the lingual tonsils. All of these tonsillar structures together are sometimes called Waldeyer's ring since they form a ring around the opening to the throat from the mouth and nose.

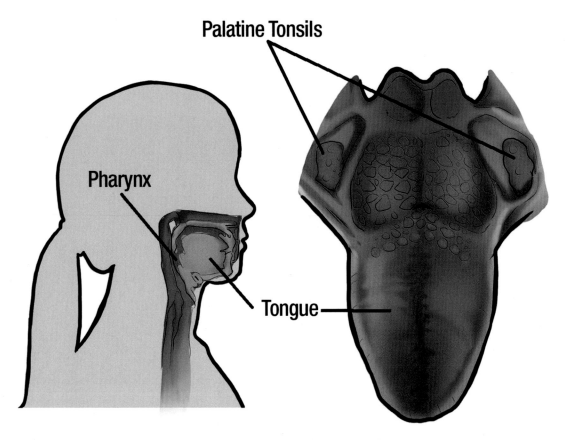

Fig. 7. The Tonsils

The tonsils are part of the lymphatic system, which helps to fight infections. However, removal of the tonsils does not seem to increase susceptibility to infection. Tonsils vary widely in size and swell in response to infection.

Mucous membranes: Mucous membranes line various cavities and canals of the organs, such as respiratory, digestive, urogenital tracts. They are equipped with innate and acquired defense mechanisms that provide a first line of defense against ingested and inhaled infectious agents. In addition, the mucosal innate immune system acts as both a physical and an immunological boundary, playing a key role in the sensing and eliminating of pathogens and in the creating of symbiosis. The mucus layer covering the mucosal epithelium acts as a first physical and biochemical barrier. An additional layer of physical protection against microorganisms is provided by a tightly interlaced cell-to-cell network of epithelial cells and intraepithelial lymphocytes.

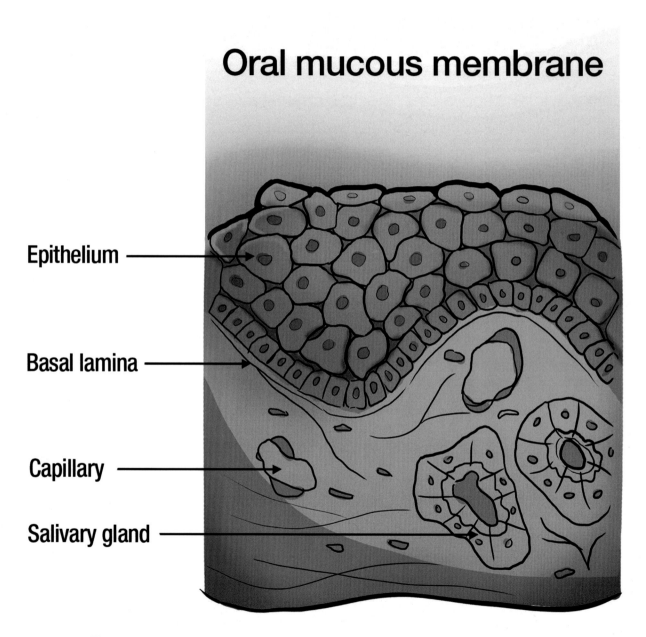

Fig 8. Mucous membrane (<u>www.health.ccm.net</u>, searched on February 8, 2022).

Various antimicrobial peptides produced by the epithelium and secreted into the mucosal lumen can directly kill the invading pathogenic bacteria. Toll-like receptors (TLRs) associated with the mucosal compartment have been shown to recognize the Pathogen-Associated Molecular Patterns (PAMPs) of a variety of pathogenic and commensal microorganisms. Therefore, a greater understanding of the immunological progression from mucosal innate to acquired immune systems should facilitate the development of new generation of mucosal vaccines to prevent and control infectious diseases.

A mucous membrane or mucosa is a membrane that lines various cavities in the body and covers the surface of internal organs. It consists of one or more layers of epithelial cells overlying a layer of loose connective tissue. It is mostly of endodermal origin and is continuous with the skin at body openings such as the eyes, ears, inside the nose, inside the mouth, lip, vagina, the urethral opening and the anus. Some mucous membranes secrete mucus, a thick protective fluid. The mucous membrane stops pathogens and dirt from entering the body and prevents bodily tissues from becoming dehydrated.

Skin: Skin as an immune organ is a protective interface between internal organs and the environment. Immune responses in the skin involve an armamentarium of immune-competent cells and soluble biologic response modifiers including cytokines. It is traversed by a network of lymphatic and blood vessels.

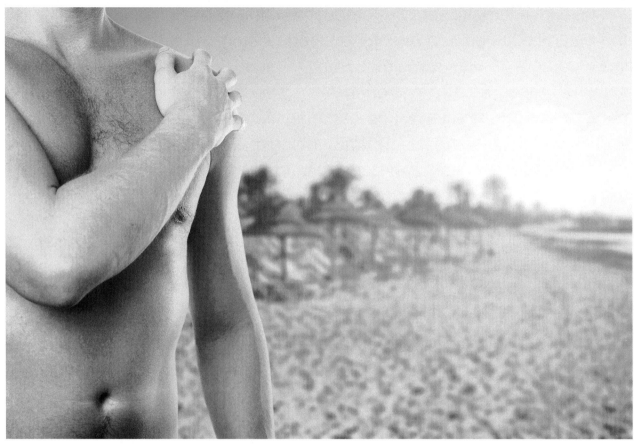

Fig 9. Skin of the body of a young man (https://bio.libretexts.org/, searched on February 8, 2022).

Skin acts as a barrier to pathogens such as viruses and microorganisms from entering the body. It is virtually impossible for them to enter through intact epidermal layers. Generally, pathogens can enter the skin only if the epidermis has been breached, for example, by a cut, puncture, or scrape. That's why it is important to clean and cover even a minor wound in the epidermis. This helps ensure that pathogens do not use the wound to enter the body. Protection from pathogens is also provided by conditions at or near the skin surface. These include relatively high acidity (pH of about 5.0), low amounts of water, antimicrobial substances produced by epidermal cells, and Langerhans cells, which phagocytize bacteria or other pathogens. The skin is an organ of the integumentary system made up of multiple layers of ectodermal tissue and guards the underlying muscles, bones, ligaments, and internal organs. Skin of a different nature exists in amphibians, reptiles, and birds. Skin plays crucial roles in formation, structure, and function of extraskeletal apparatus. The dermis contains most of the lymphocytes in the skin, other migrant leukocytes, mast cells, and tissue macrophages.

The key immune cells in the epidermis are epidermal dendritic cells (Langerhans cells) and keratinocytes.

The dermis has blood and lymph vessels and numerous immune cells, including dermal dendritic cells, lymphocytes—T cells, B cells, natural killer (NK) cells, and mast cells.

There is continuous trafficking of immune cells between the skin, draining lymph nodes, and blood circulation.

CHAPTER 5

☺VACCINES

"A vaccine is a biological preparation given to stimulate the body's production of antibodies and provide immunity against a disease" (www.fda.gov, 2021).

A vaccine is made from a very small amount of attenuated or inactivated disease-causing organisms or their genetic material. A vaccinated person can fight the disease faster and more effectively and stop the disease from happening. Vaccines play an important role in keeping us healthy. They protect us from serious and sometimes deadly diseases. All vaccines work by exposing the body to molecules from the target pathogen to trigger an immune response.

Vaccination is the act of getting a vaccine, usually as a shot.

Immunization can also mean the process of getting vaccinated. Immunization fortifies an individual's immune system against an infectious agent (the immunogen). Immunization is an adaptive immune system.

Getting vaccinated with the COVID-19 vaccine (now available from several pharmaceutical companies) is the best hope for ending the pandemic (fig. 1).

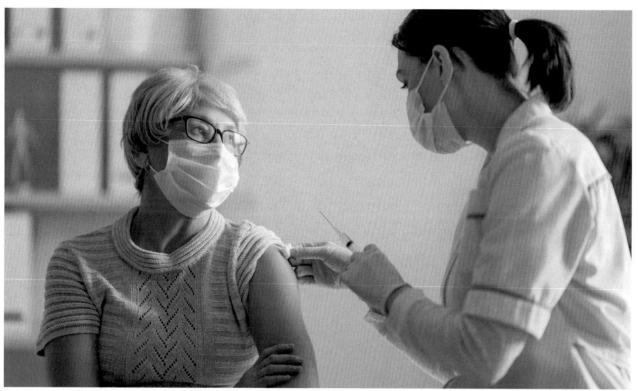

Fig. 1. Nurse gives senior adult healthcare worker the COVID-19 vaccine
(https://www.gettyimages.com/, searched on February 9, 2022).

"Immunization is one of modern medicine's greatest success stories. Time and again, the international community has endorsed the value of vaccines and immunization to prevent and control a large number of infectious diseases, such as pneumonia, measles, polio, whooping cough, etc." (https://www.who.int, 2021).

Vaccines have protected people against a variety of diseases.

Vaccines against Diseases

Measles, mumps, rubella (MMR) vaccine. Measles, mumps, and rubella are all viral, contagious diseases that can be prevented by a single vaccination (known as the MMR vaccine).

Here are some details about the three diseases:

Measles. "Measles is caused by Measles virus, also called Morbilivirus, member of Paramyxoviridae family" ((https://viralzone.expasy.org/678, 2021).

In the early 1960s, over half a million children were infected every year. In 1963, the creation of a measles vaccine changed everything. Today, while very few new cases of measles occur each year in developed countries, it still occurs in epidemic proportions in developing regions, infecting around 20 million people and causing around 140,000 deaths worldwide.

Mumps. "Mumps is caused by mumps virus, also called rubulavirus, member of Paramyxoviridae family" ((https://viralzone.expasy.org/678, 2021).

Rubella. "Rubella is caused by rubella virus, also called rubivirus, member of Togaviridae family" (https://viralzone.expasy.org/678, 2021).

In spite of MMR vaccination, children with perinatal human immunodeficiency virus (HIV) infection (PHIV) may not be protected against measles, mumps, and rubella because of impaired initial vaccine response or waning immunity (Siberry et al. 2015).

Earlier work on vaccine development. In the 1940s, a combination diphtheria-tetanus-pertussis vaccine was introduced as DTwP. It contained diphtheria toxin, tetanus toxin, and whole (but killed) *Bordetella pertussis* bacteria. By the mid-1970s, however, due to adverse reactions attributed to the whole-cell vaccine, some patients and parents began to reject the vaccine despite the continuing circulation of *B. pertussis* and pertussis disease. As vaccination rates went down, infection rates crept up. To address these issues, the National Institutes of Health held an international symposium to examine the risks and benefits of whole-cell pertussis vaccination in November 1978.

Pertussis, also known as whooping cough, is a highly contagious respiratory disease. Pertussis is known for uncontrollable, violent coughing which often makes it hard to breathe. After cough fits, someone with pertussis often needs to take deep breaths, which result in a "whooping" sound. Pertussis can affect people of all ages but can be very serious, even deadly, for babies less than a year old.

In the 1970s and 1980s, John J. "Jack" Muñoz and his colleagues at National Institute of Allergy and Infectious Diseases (NIAID) Rocky Mountain Laboratories made key discoveries about these bacterial components and their role in inducing immunity to pertussis. In 1986, Dr. Muñoz's group successfully isolated and characterized a fragment of *B. pertussis* DNA containing the genes for pertussis toxin, the substance responsible for establishing infection, and mapped these genes within the bacterial genome. 1996 licensure and use of the first diphtheria-tetanus-acellular pertussis

(DTaP) vaccine in the United States. Today, the Centers for Disease Control and Prevention (CDC) recommend the DTaP vaccine for infants and children (NIH-NIAID, 2021).

Vaccines available today. Today we have vaccines against more than 25 different diseases. Here we mention some of them: adenovirus, anthrax, BCG, cholera, COVID-19, dengue, diphtheria, Ebola, hemophilis, hepatitis, influenza, measles, meningococcal, mumps, plaque, pneumococcal, papilloma, polio, rabies, rotavirus, rubella, smallpox, tetanus, yellow fever, and zoster (https://www.who.int, 2021).

Classification of vaccines: There are four basic types of vaccines.

Whole virus vaccines

Nucleic acid vaccines

Protein subunit vaccines

Viral vector-based vaccines

Whole virus vaccines:

Whole virus vaccines use a weakened (attenuated) or deactivated form of the pathogen that causes a disease to trigger protective immunity to it. There are two types of whole virus vaccines. **Live attenuated** vaccines use a weakened form of the virus, which can still grow and replicate, but does not cause illness.

Inactivated vaccines contain viruses whose genetic material has been destroyed by heat, chemicals or radiation so they cannot infect cells and replicate, but can still trigger an immune response.

The live attenuated vaccines are derived from "wild" viruses or bacteria. These wild viruses or bacteria are attenuated (weakened) in a laboratory, usually by repeated culturing. For example, the measles virus used as a vaccine today was isolated from a child with measles disease in 1954. Almost 10 years of serial passage using tissue culture media were required to transform the wild virus into the attenuated vaccine virus. To produce an immune response, live, attenuated vaccines must replicate in the vaccinated person. A relatively small dose of administered virus or bacteria replicates in the body and creates enough of the organism to stimulate an immune response. Although live, attenuated vaccines replicate, they usually do not cause disease such as that caused by the wild form of the organism. When a live, attenuated vaccine does cause disease, it is usually much milder than the natural disease and is considered an adverse reaction to the vaccine. The immune response to a live, attenuated vaccine is virtually identical to that produced by a natural infection because the immune system does not differentiate between an infection with a weakened vaccine virus and an infection with a wild virus. Injected live, attenuated vaccines produce immunity in most recipients with one dose. However, a small percentage of recipients do not respond to the first dose of an injected live, attenuated vaccine (such as measles, mumps, and rubella [MMR]) and a second dose is recommended to provide an extremely high level of immunity in the population. Orally administered live, attenuated vaccines require more than one dose to produce immunity. A live, attenuated vaccine may cause severe or fatal infections as a result of uncontrolled replication of the vaccine virus or bacteria. However, this only occurs in persons with a weakened immune system (e.g., from leukemia, treatment with certain drugs, or human immunodeficiency virus [HIV] infection). A live, attenuated vaccine virus could theoretically revert to its original pathogenic form. For this reason, they are considered not safe. (https://www.who.int, 2021).

Inactivated vaccines contain viruses whose genetic material has been destroyed. Inactivated vaccines are derived from inactivated whole cells (e.g., polio, hepatitis A, and rabies vaccines), subunits (e.g., influenza and pneumococcal vaccines), toxoids (e.g., diphtheria and tetanus toxoid), and recombinant molecules (e.g., hepatitis B, human papillomavirus [HPV], and influenza [Flublok brand]). The genetic material is inactivated by heat, chemicals or radiation so they cannot infect cells and replicate, but can still trigger an immune response. Even though their genetic material has been destroyed, inactivated viruses usually contain many proteins which the immune system can react to. But because they cannot infect cells, inactivated vaccines only stimulate antibody-mediated responses, and this response may be weaker and less long-lived. To overcome this problem, inactivated vaccines are often given alongside adjuvants (agents that stimulate the immune system).

Both attenuated and inactivated vaccine strategies form the basis of many existing vaccines – including yellow fever and measles (live attenuated vaccines), or seasonal influenza and hepatitis A (inactivated vaccines). Bacterial attenuated vaccines also exist, such as the BCG vaccine for tuberculosis. Bacillus Calmette–Guérin (BCG) vaccine is a vaccine primarily used against tuberculosis. It is named after its inventors Albert Calmette and Camille Guérin. In countries where TB or leprosy is common, one dose is recommended in healthy babies as soon after birth as possible (https://en.wikipedia.org/, 2021).

Because these vaccines are simply weakened versions of natural pathogens, the immune system responds as it would to any other cellular invader. The immune system mobilizes a range of defenses against it, including killer T cells (which identify and destroy infected cells), helper T cells (which support antibody production), antibody-producing B cells, and the memory cells. Thus, the vaccines can trigger an immune response which is almost as good as being exposed to the wild virus, but without falling ill.

Nucleic acid vaccines: These include DNA and RNA vaccines.

Nucleic acid vaccines: Nucleic acid vaccines, DNA, and messenger RNA (mRNA) that codes for the proteins that pathogens use to cause disease. These vaccines enable the body to innately mimic a native infection to elicit an immune response, but without the ability to cause disease or spread. Once the DNA or RNA is inside the cell and it starts producing antigens, these are then displayed on its surface, where they can be detected by the immune system, triggering a response. This response includes killer T cells, which seek out and destroy infected cells, as well as antibody-producing B cells and helper T cells which support antibody production.

DNA vaccines: Deoxyribonucleic acid (DNA) is the genetic material, the main constituent of the chromosomes, present in the nucleus of the cells. It has a unique double-helix shape, like a twisted ladder. It contains 4 basic building blocks or bases—adenine (A), cytosine (C), guanine (G), and thymine (T), which make the genetic code.

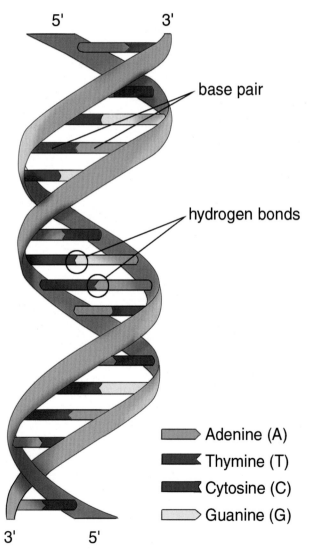

base pair

hydrogen bonds

Adenine (A)
Thymine (T)
Cytosine (C)
Guanine (G)

Fig. 2. An illustration to show the double helix structure of DNA (image credit: Genome Research

Limited, https://www.yourgenome.org, searched on February 9, 2022).

DNA vaccines contain a piece of DNA encoding the antigen. This is a circular piece of DNA, called plasmid used by bacteria to store and share genes which may benefit their survival. Plasmids can replicate independently of the main chromosomal DNA and provide a simple tool for transferring genes between cells. Because of this, they are widely used in the field of genetic engineering.

Plasmids: *Plasmids are double-stranded, generally circular DNA sequences capable of automatically replicating in a host cell. Plasmid vectors minimally consist of the transgene insert and an origin of replication, which allows for semi-independent replication of the plasmid in the host. Modern plasmids generally have many more features, notably a "multiple cloning site", with nucleotide overhangs for insertion of an insert and multiple restriction enzyme consensus sites on either side of the insert (fig. 3).*

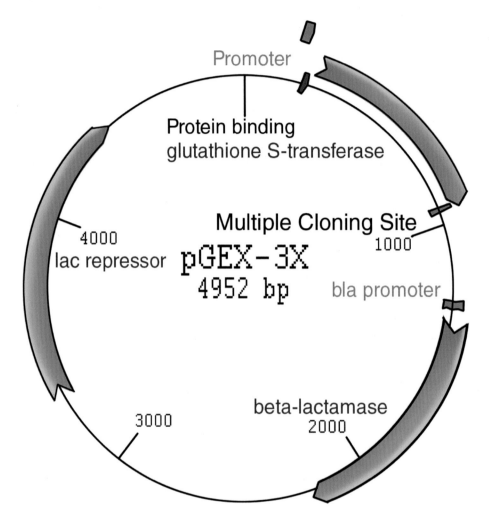

Fig. 3. The pGEX-3x plasmid is a popular cloning vector. The various elements of the plasmid are labeled (https://bio.libretexts.org/, searched on February 9, 2022).

Plasmid vaccine: DNA vaccines work by injecting genetically engineered plasmid containing the DNA sequence encoding the antigen(s) against which an immune response is sought, so the cells directly produce the antigen, thus causing a protective immunological response.

There are different types of vaccines, which can be grouped into three categories (M. Zahn, A. Serwer, 2022).

First-generation vaccines make use of the entire virus weakened or attenuated. Examples of first-generation vaccines are measles, mumps, rubella, polio, hepatitis, and rabies.

Second-generation vaccines use specific viral proteins or protein fragments instead of a whole virus. Examples of second-generation vaccines are hepatitis B and human papillomavirus (HPV).

Third-generation vaccines use specific viral genes or viral RNA that encode the desired viral protein. Examples of third-generation vaccines are COVID-19and adenovirus. Both Pfizer and Moderna pharmaceutical companies use viral RNA to make vaccines.

RNA vaccines: RNA vaccines encode the antigen of interest in messenger RNA (mRNA) or self-amplifying RNA (saRNA)—molecular templates used by cellular factories to produce proteins. Because of its transitory nature, there is zero risk of it integrating with our own genetic material. The RNA can be injected by itself, encapsulated within nanoparticles (as Pfizer's mRNA-based COVID vaccine is), or driven into cells using some of the same techniques being developed for DNA vaccines.

mRNA is a single-stranded nucleic acid molecule that carries genetic sequence from the DNA inside the cell's nucleus and comes out of the nucleus in the cellular cytoplasm where it is translated into the protein.

When DNA in a gene is transcribed, it produces RNA transcript, called messenger RNA.

An illustration showing the process of transcription.

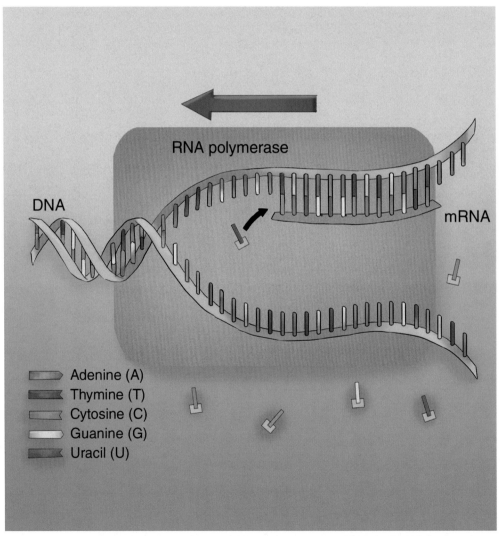

Fig. 4. Process of biosynthesis from DNA to messenger RNA (mRNA) (Image credit: Genome Research Limited, https://www.yourgenome.org/, searched on February 9, 2022).

Messenger ribonucleic acid (mRNA) is a single-stranded molecule of RNA that corresponds to the genetic sequence of a gene and is read by a ribosome in the process of synthesizing a protein.

The process, known as in-vitro transcription, can generate many mRNA molecules from a strand of DNA in a test tube. This requires an enzyme (called RNA polymerase) and nucleotides (the molecules that are the building blocks of DNA and RNA). When mixed together, the polymerase reads the strand of DNA and converts the code into a strand of mRNA, by linking different nucleotides together in the correct order.

The RNA sequence used in the COVID-19 vaccine developed by Pfizer and BioNTech is a modified form of the Uridine nucleotide (U), referred as pseudo uridine (Ψ) (M. D. Buchamann et al. 2021). RNA vaccine developed by Moderna Pharmaceuticals as well as Pfizer and BioNTech Co., contain modified RNA and lipid nanoparticles.

INSIDE AN MRNA COVID VACCINE

COVID-19 vaccines made from messenger RNA use lipid nanoparticles — bubbles of fats — to carry molecules into cells. The mRNA contains the code for cells to produce the 'spike' protein that the coronavirus SARS-CoV-2 uses to enter cells. Here are key innovations in the design of these vaccines

mRNA

CGAGΨΨCGΨGΨΨΨAA

The vaccines made by Moderna and Pfizer-BioNTech use mRNA that has been chemically modified to replace the uridine (U) nucleotide with pseudouridine (Ψ).
This change is thought to stop the immune system reacting to the introduced mRNA.

To help the body mount an effective immune response to later SARS-CoV-2 infections, the mRNA sequence is adapted to stabilize the spike protein in the shape it used when fusing with human cells

Lipid nanoparticle

Lipids

Phospholipid
Cholesterol
Ionizable lipid
PEG-lipid*

The fatty nanoparticle around the mRNA is made of four types of lipid molecule. One of these is 'ionizable': in the vaccine, many of these molecules have a positive charge and cling to negatively charged mRNA, but they lose that charge in the more alkaline conditions of the bloodstream, reducing toxicity in the body.

*Lipid attached to polyethylene glycol

Nik Spencer/*Nature*, adapted from M. D. Buschmann *et al. Vaccines* **9**, 65 (2021)
Fig. 5. COVID-19 vaccine made from modified mRNA that gets translated into the spike protein (M. D. Buschmann et al. 2021).

Protein subunit vaccines:

The mRNA is translated into the protein, by the process, translation. It occurs in the ribosomes of the cell. Transfer RNA (tRNA) carries an amino acid to mRNA, and the mRNA is read three bases (a codon). Each codon specifies a particular amino acid. For example, the three bases GGU code for amino acid, glycine. There are 64 combinations of codon for 20 amino acids. Each amino acid is attached specifically to its own tRNA molecule. When the mRNA sequence is read, each tRNA molecule delivers its amino acid to the ribosome and binds temporarily to the corresponding codon on the mRNA molecule. Once the tRNA is bound, it releases its amino acid and the adjacent amino acids all join together into a long chain, called a polypeptide. This process continues until protein is formed.

Protein subunit vaccines are produced by chemically attaching a polysaccharide from the surface of bacteria to a protein molecule through a process called conjugation. Conjugating a polysaccharide antigen to a protein molecule produces long-lasting protective immunity to the polysaccharide antigen (e.g., Haemophilus influenzae type b and pneumococcal conjugate vaccines).

The immune response to a pure polysaccharide vaccine is typically T-cell-independent, which means these vaccines can stimulate B-cells without the assistance of T-helper cells. T-cell-independent antigens, including polysaccharide vaccines, are not consistently immunogenic in children younger than age 2 years, probably because of immaturity of the immune system. Attaching the polysaccharide antigen to a protein makes it possible to prevent bacterial infections in populations where a polysaccharide vaccine is not effective or provides only temporary protection.

Rather than injecting a whole pathogen to trigger an immune response, subunit vaccines (sometimes called acellular vaccines) contain purified pieces of it, which have been specially selected for their ability to stimulate immune cells. Because these fragments are incapable of causing disease, subunit vaccines are considered very safe. There are several types: protein subunit vaccines contain specific isolated proteins from viral or bacterial pathogens; polysaccharide vaccines contain chains of sugar molecules (polysaccharides) found in the cell walls of some bacteria; conjugate subunit vaccines bind a polysaccharide chain to a carrier protein to try and boost the immune response. Only protein subunit vaccines are being developed against the virus that causes COVID-19.

Other subunit vaccines are already in widespread use. Examples include the hepatitis B and acellular pertussis vaccines (protein subunit), the pneumococcal polysaccharide vaccine (polysaccharide), and the MenACWY vaccine, which contains polysaccharides from the surface of four types of the bacteria which causes meningococcal disease joined to diphtheria or tetanus toxoid (conjugate subunit).

Protein subunit vaccines contain fragments of protein and/or polysaccharide from the pathogen, which have been carefully studied to identify which combinations of these molecules are likely to produce a strong and effective immune response. By restricting the immune system's access to the pathogen in this way, the risk of side effects is minimized. Such vaccines are also relatively cheap and easy to produce, and more stable than those containing whole viruses or bacteria.

A downside of this precision is that the antigens used to elicit an immune response may lack molecular structures called pathogen-associated molecular patterns which are common to a class of pathogen. These structures can be read by immune cells and recognized as danger signals, so their absence may result in a weaker immune response. Also, because the antigens do not infect cells, subunit vaccines mainly only trigger antibody-mediated immune responses. Again, this means the immune response may be weaker than with other types of vaccines. To overcome this problem, subunit vaccines are sometimes delivered alongside adjuvants (agents that stimulate the immune system).

All subunit vaccines are made using living organisms, such as bacteria and yeast, which require substrates on which to grow them, and strict hygiene to avoid contamination with other organisms. This makes them more expensive to produce than chemically-synthesized vaccines, such as RNA vaccines. (https://www.gavi.org/vaccineswork/, searched on February 12, 2022)

The precise manufacturing method depends on the type of subunit vaccine being produced. Protein subunit vaccines, such as the recombinant hepatitis B vaccine, are made by inserting the genetic code for the antigen into yeast cells, which are relatively easy to grow and capable of synthesizing large amounts of protein. The yeast is grown in large fermentation tanks, and then split open, allowing the antigen to be harvested. This purified protein is then added to other vaccine components, such as preservatives to keep it stable, and adjuvants to boost the immune response – in this case alum. For polysaccharide or conjugate vaccines, the polysaccharide is produced by growing bacteria in industrial bioreactors, before splitting them open and harvesting the polysaccharide from their cell walls. In the case of conjugate vaccines, the protein that the polysaccharide is attached to must also be prepared by growing a different type of bacteria in separate bioreactors. Once its proteins are harvested, they are chemically attached to the polysaccharide, and then the remaining vaccine components added. (Source)

Viral vector-based vaccines: Various viruses have been developed as vectors, including adenovirus (a cause of the common cold), measles virus, and vaccinia virus. These vectors are stripped of any disease-causing genes and sometimes also genes that can enable them to replicate, meaning they are now harmless. The genetic instructions for making the antigen from the target pathogen are stitched into the virus vector's genome.

Viral vector vaccines: The Oxford/AstraZeneca coronavirus vaccine used the viral vector approach. The genetic sequence of adenovirus, a pathogen that causes common cold, was spliced into the genetic sequence from the coronavirus. The adenovirus simply serves as the vehicle to get the genetic sequence of coronavirus into the human cells. That's why it's called a viral vector.

Viral vector vaccines use a harmless virus to deliver a piece of genetic code to the human cells, allowing them to make a pathogen's protein. This trains our immune system to react to future infections.

The harmless virus acts as a delivery system, or vector, for the genetic sequence. Our cells then make the viral or bacterial protein that the vector has delivered and present it to our immune system. This allows us to develop a specific immune response against a pathogen without the need to have an infection.

However, the viral vector itself plays an additional role by boosting our immune response. This leads to a more robust reaction than if the pathogen's genetic sequence was delivered on its own.

The Oxford-AstraZeneca COVID-19 vaccine uses a chimpanzee common cold viral vector known as ChAdOx1, which delivers the code that allows our cells to make the SARS-CoV-2 spike protein. Our cells then transcribe this gene into messenger RNA, or mRNA, which in turn prompts our cellular machine to make the spike protein in the main body, or the cytoplasm, of the cell.

Then our cells present the spike protein, as well as small parts of it, on the cell surface, prompting our immune system to make antibodies and mount T cell responses. Researchers have shown that this vaccine is effective in preventing SARS-CoV-2 infection. (https://www.gavi.org/vaccineswork/, searched on February 12, 2022).

Vaccines for COVID-19: Vaccines are now available to prevent the COVID-19 disease pandemic.

U.S. Food and Drug Administration (FDA) has approved and authorized the use of a few COVID-19 vaccines.

Moderna Therapeutics Company (Cambridge, MA 02139, USA) uses mRNA-based vaccine technology. The mRNA offers us a new paradigm in vaccination as these vaccines work seamlessly with the body to mimic the natural sequence of exposure and protection, without the dangers of a real infection (K Bahl et al. 2017, Moderna Therapeutics Company).

Effectiveness of the vaccines with COVID-19 variants: The coronavirus is all encoded on a single mRNA, the variants may not pose any big threat to the effectiveness of vaccines. The variations could require annual modifications. A clinical trial was conducted to determine whether people who are highly allergic or have a mast cell disorder are at increased risk for allergic reactions to the Moderna or Pfizer-BioNTech COVID-19 vaccines (NIAID, NIH, 2020). The authorities and the people will be evaluating the benefits and the side effects of these vaccines. There is a dire need for these vaccines as long as the infection continues (K. Bahl et al. 2017, Moderna Therapeutics Company).

Manufacturing and Distribution of COVID Vaccine: Operation Warp Speed (OWS) aims to deliver 300 million doses of a safe, effective vaccine for COVID-19 by Jan 2021, as a part of a broader strategy to accelerate the development, manufacturing, and distribution of COVID-19 vaccines, therapeutics, and diagnostics (collectively known as countermeasures) (Food and Drug Administration, USA, 2021).

Measures taken by the US government to combat the COVID-19 pandemic:

The policy tracker, issued by International Monetary Fund (www.imf.org) summarizes the key economic responses governments are taking to limit the human and economic impact of the Global COVID-19 Pandemic. The United States government is working with the United Nations Security Council and with partners to strengthen multilateral public health and humanitarian cooperation on the COVID-19 response, global institutions to combat disease, and global health security architecture to prevent, detect, and respond to future biological threats.

Global COVID-19 Summit: Ending the Pandemic and Building Back Better. "On September 22, 2021, President Joe Biden convened a virtual Global COVID-19 Summit focused on ending the pandemic and building better health security to prevent and prepare for future biological threats. The President called on the world to collectively end the COVID-19 pandemic as soon as possible, with every country, partner, and organization doing its part, aligning around shared goals and targets, and holding each other to account. At the same time, all countries need the capacity to prevent, detect, and respond to biological threats, including future pandemics. The Summit introduced ambitious targets in three critical areas for ending this pandemic and preventing and preparing for the next: **Vaccinate the World**; **Save Lives Now**; and **Build Back Better**" (Statements and Releases, www.whitehouse.gov/briefing-room/, 2021).

President Biden rolls up his sleeve for a booster shot of the coronavirus vaccine.

Pres. Joseph R. Biden received a booster shot of Pfizer's coronavirus vaccine. President Biden said, "Let me be clear, boosters are important, but the most important thing we need to do is get more people vaccinated."

References Vaccines:

Bahl, K., Senn, J. J., Yuzhakov, O., et al. 2017. "Preclinical and Clinical Demonstration of Immunogenicity by mRNA Vaccines against H10N8 and H7N9 Influenza Viruses, Mol Therapy" 25(6):1316–1338. http://dx.doi.org/10.1016/j.ymthe.2017.03.035.

Buschmann, M. D., Carrasco, M. J., Alishetty, S., et al. 2021. "Nanomaterial delivery systems for mRNA vaccines." *Vaccines* 9(1): 65. https://doi.org/10.3390/vaccines9010065.

Contreras, Oliver for *The Washington Post*. 2021.

Ghaffarifar, F. "Plasmid DNA vaccines: where are we now?" *Drugs Today* (Barc). 2018. (May) 54(5):315-333. doi: 10.1358/dot.2018.54.5.2807864. PMID: 29911696.

Siberry, G. K., Patel, K., Bellini, W. J., et al. 2015. "Pediatric HIV AIDS Cohort Study PHACS. Immunity to Measles, Mumps, and Rubella in US Children With Perinatal HIV Infection or Perinatal HIV Exposure Without Infection." *Clinical Infectious Diseases*. (Sep. 15, 2015) 61(6):988-95. doi: 10.1093/cid/civ440. Epub 2015 Jun 9. PMID: 26060291; PMCID: PMC4551008.

"Statements and Releases 2021 Global COVID-19 Summit: Ending the Pandemic and Building Back Better." www.whitehouse.gov/briefing-room/.

Zahn, M., Serwer, A. 2022. "Second and third generation COVID vaccines are coming." (Jan. 28, 2022) www.news.yahoo.com.

2021. https://en.wikipedia.org/.

2021. fda.usa.gov.

https://www.gavi.org/vaccineswork/, searched February 12, 2022.

https://www.gettyimages.com/, searched on February 9, 2022.

NIH: National Institute of Allergy and Infectious Diseases. "Leading research to understand, treat, and prevent infectious, immunologic, and allergic diseases." 2021.

https://viralzone.expasy.org/678, 2021.

https://www.hhs.gov/immunization/basics/index.html.

https://www.who.int, 2021.

https://www.who.int/immunization/documents/Elsevier Vaccine immunology.pdf

www.yalemedicine.org/news/vaccine-basics

https://en.wikipedia.org/, 2021.

CHAPTER 6

ATTEMPTS TO DEVELOP DRUGS TO CURE SARS-COV-2

Attempts are being made to test chemical compounds with antiviral activity to find treatments for SARS-CoV-2 infected patients.

Scientific databases reported on treatment and management of viruses from various resources; Google search, Pubmed, NCBI, Research Gate, etc., are being analyzed in order to identify the medicinal agents as a treatment for COVID-19.

Research is being focused on new as well as existing antiviral drugs that could be used with adequate safety and effective monitoring protocols.

Fighting the COVID-19 pandemic is a top priority in medical research and pharmaceutical development. Hundreds of organizations are working on innovations to reduce the impact of SARS-CoV-2 and prevent further infection.

After the discussion on vaccines that have been developed to prevent and slow down the spread of the virus, we are going to discuss in this chapter therapies and drugs for treatments for people that have caught the virus and suffering from its deadly and horrible consequences.

How do clinicians assess and incorporate information on treating a potentially fatal new disease? The COVID-19 pandemic brought this question into focus as rapidly emerging evidence-informed decisions on implementing and de-implementing treatments.

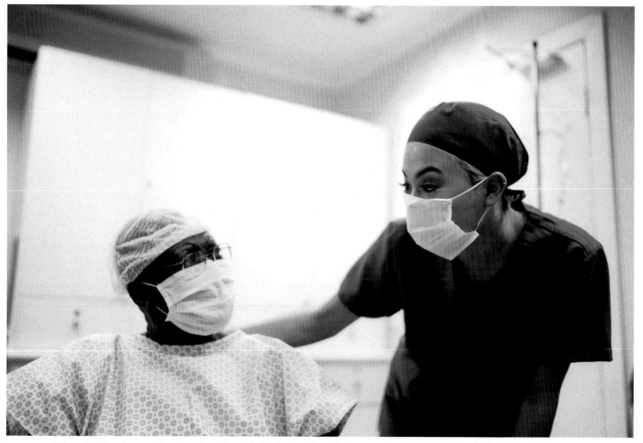

Fig. 1. The important role of antivirals in the fight against COVID-19 (R. Moscicki, 2021).

Antivirals are molecules specifically created to target the virus directly, disrupting or stopping its ability to replicate and spread.

Hundreds of clinical trials are currently investigating antivirals for COVID-19, including more than a dozen newly developed antivirals specifically designed to target the SARS-CoV-2 virus (R. Moscicki R, 2021).

Traditionally, peer-reviewed, published, randomized clinical trials define the standard of care for treatment. In the setting of COVID-19, a more rapid response evolved; available drugs were repurposed for treatment on the basis of in vitro data, anecdotal reports, case series, and retrospective observational studies because of desperation to "do something." This was fueled by colleagues, patients and their families, the popular press, and social media led to a cacophony of treatment approaches.

An extreme example occurred early in pandemic when hydroxychloroquine plus azithromycin were initially declared on March 21, 2020, as a real chance to be the biggest game changers in the history of medicine. Ultimately, clinical trials failed to demonstrate benefit (M. J., Glesby, 2021).

COVID-19 is an infectious disease; the treatment for COVID-19 depends on the severity of the infection.

For milder illnesses, resting at home and taking medicine to reduce fever is often sufficient.

For more severe cases, assisted oxygen and other supportive measures are required, so hospitalization becomes necessary.

Federal Drug Administration (USA) has approved antiviral drugs and therapies for the treatment of hospitalized patients with COVID-19.

FDA has given authorization for the use of convalescent blood plasma therapy (CBPT).

Convalescent blood plasma therapy: When people become infected and ill from a virus and then get better (convalesce), their immune system has successfully produced antibodies to fight that virus. Doctors have used forms of antibody therapy for over a hundred years in medical treatment.

Antiviral drugs for COVID-19 treatment: Effective antiviral treatments can shorten the duration of the illness and lessen complications in some people. Since the coronavirus that causes COVID-19 is new, there is limited evidence regarding specific anti-viral that may work against it. Doctors and scientists are looking at experimental anti-viral to find effective treatments for the new disease.

There are several anti-viral drugs that are being used for COVID-19 treatment:

1. remdesivir

2. molnupiravir/ EIDD-2801

3. ritonavir/Norvir

4. dexamethasone

5. interferons

1. **Remdesivir for COVID-19 treatment**: Remdesivir, antiviral drug, was initially developed for the Ebola virus treatment. Ebola virus caused deadly infection that led to profuse internal and external bleeding and eventually led to organ failure.

Remdesivir is a nucleoside analog with a broad antiviral activity spectrum among RNA viruses, including Ebola virus (EBOV) and the respiratory pathogens. First described in 2016, the drug was derived from an antiviral library of small molecules intended to target emerging pathogenic RNA viruses. *In vivo*, remdesivir showed therapeutic and prophylactic effects in animal models of EBOV, MERS-CoV, SARS-CoV, and SARS-CoV-2 infection. However, the substance failed in a clinical trial on Ebola virus disease (EVD), where it was inferior to investigational monoclonal antibodies in an interim analysis. As there was no placebo control in this study, no conclusions on its efficacy in EVD can be made. In contrast, data from a placebo-controlled trial show beneficial effects for patients with COVID-19. Remdesivir reduced the time to recovery of hospitalized patients who required supplemental oxygen and may have a positive impact on mortality outcomes while having a favorable safety profile.

Remdesivir is a monophosphoramidate nucleoside prodrug that undergoes intracellular metabolic conversion to its active metabolite nucleoside triphosphate (NTP).

The National Institutes of Health reported that in a US clinical trial (ACTT-1), remdesivir helped patients with COVID-19 recover faster when compared with patients who did not receive the drug

Mechanism of action: Remdesivir is an inhibitor of the SARS-CoV-2 RNA-dependent RNA polymerase (RdRp), which is essential for viral replication.

2. Molnupiravir/ EIDD-2801 (chemical name is **EIDD-2801) for COVID-19 treatment:** Molnupiravir forces the SARS-CoV-2 coronavirus to mutate itself to death.

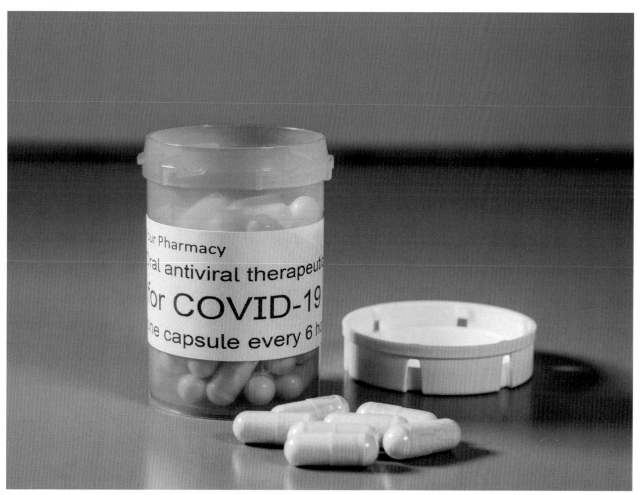

Fig. 2. Molnupiravir/ EIDD-2801for treatment for COVID-19 (Credit: Merck & Co Inc/Handout/*Reuters*)

Molnupiravir/ **EIDD-2801** was so effective in a phase 3 trial involving COVID-19-positive people at risk of severe illness that clinicians halted enrolment early. But whether this clinical-trial success story will translate into a global game-changer in the fight against the pandemic isn't yet clear.

Drug Innovation Ventures at Emory (DRIVE) tested molnupiravir as possible therapy for Venezuelan equine encephalitis. Next they discovered that it worked against mouse hepatitis virus, MERS, and coronaviruses. It silenced the virus's ability to replicate, and also suppressed the virus's transmission from infected to uninfected participants.

Administration and dosage: As EIDD-2801 is still in an experimental stage, doses of 200–800 mg administered orally every 12 hours for 5 days were tested (A. Wahl et al. 2021).

Mechanism of action: EIDD-2801 acts as a competitive alternate substrate for the viral RNA-dependent RNA polymerase, which allows the incorporation of 5′-triphosphate into viral RNA and results in the accumulation of mutations within the viral RNA genome that lead to error catastrophe. EIDD-2801, an oral broad-spectrum antiviral markedly inhibited SARS-CoV-2 replication in vivo, and thus has considerable potential for the prevention and treatment of COVID-19.

3. Ritonavir/Norvir: Ritonavir (brand name Norvir) is a prescription medicine approved by the U.S. Food and Drug Administration (FDA) for the treatment of HIV infection in adults and children older than 1 month. Ritonavir is always used in combination with other HIV medicines. Although ritonavir is FDA-approved for the treatment of HIV infection, it is no longer used for its activity against HIV. Instead, ritonavir (given at low doses) is currently used as a pharmacokinetic enhancer to boost the activity of other HIV medicines.

Ritonavir belongs to a class of drugs known as protease inhibitors. It increases («boosts») the levels of other protease inhibitors, which helps these medications work better (https://www.webmd.com/, searched February 13, 2022).

4. Dexamethasone for COVID-19 treatment: Dexamethasone is a glucocorticoid (steroid), a medication to treat rheumatic problems, arthritis, inflammation, asthma, chronic obstructive lung disease, eye pain following eye surgery, and along with antibiotics in tuberculosis.

For COVID-19 patients, dexamethasone combats inflammation of the lungs and other organs, and it improves survival of the hospitalized patients requiring oxygen. Among the scores of potential therapies studied in clinical trials aimed at improving the treatment of COVID-19, dexamethasone was a home run. Its subsequent fast adoption and usage in the vast majority of patients who might stand to benefit is actually a "testament to how clinicians have been able to keep up with the avalanche of data, and do what's best for patients." (M. J. Glesby, 2021).

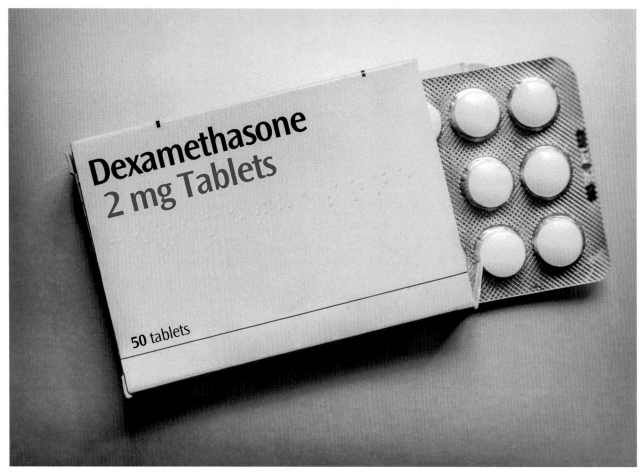

Fig. 3. Dexamethasone is a synthetic glucocorticoid (steroid)
(*Image credit:* Joshimerbin/Shutterstock.com).

Dexamethasone is the first drug shown to save lives and proved as a Coronavirus breakthrough.

Dexamethasone is a synthetic corticosteroid. When the body is stressed, corticosteroids and other hormones are released to regulate our stress response, just as insulin regulates blood sugar levels. These corticosteroids perform a huge number of tasks when released; they modulate the immune response, inflammation in the body, metabolism, blood electrolyte levels, and even behavior.

Dexamethasone has been around for decades, meaning it has been rigorously tested and implemented in medicine and is considered a reliable, low-risk medication.

Dexamethasone is manufactured globally under many trademarks as shown in table 1.

Table 1. Top Dexamethasone Manufacturers in the USA and Globally (www. marketwatch.com, 2020; https://www.thomasnet.com, 2020)

Company	Headquarters	Year Founded	Annual Sales, $
Pfizer	New York, NY	1849	52 Bill
Novartis	Basel, Switzerland	1996	49.9 Bill
Merck & Co	Kenilworth, NJ	1891	46.8 Bill
Sanofi Pharma	Paris, France	1973	40 Bill
Baxter International	Deerfield, IL	1931	11.5 Bill
Zidus Cadila	Ahmedabad, India	1951	3 Bill
Endo International	Dublin, Ireland	1997	3 Bill
Aspen Pharma	Durban, S. Africa	1850	2.8 Bill
Hikma Pharma	London, UK	1978	2.2 Bill
Cipla Ltd	Mumbai, India	1935	2.3 Bill
Wockhardt Ltd	Mumbai, India	1999	1 Bill
Xspire Pharma	Madison, MS	2011	Private
Fera Pharma	Locust Valley, NY	2009	Private
Ache Lab	Guaruhos Brazil	1966	Private
WraSer Pharma	Rigeland, MS	2002	Private

Administration and dosage of dexamethasone: Dexamethasone has recently become interesting to healthcare workers treating COVID-19, as a 2020 randomized controlled clinical trial of 2100 participants. It was concluded that six milligrams of dexamethasone per day reduced risk of dying by 20% in critically ill patients. The trial also showed that the drug had no effect on mild COVID-19 cases. This makes intuitive sense, as the severe inflammation of vital organs (lungs, heart, brain, etc.) caused by the body's response to COVID-19 seems to be the leading cause of coronavirus deaths. People only mildly sick may not benefit from such a reduction, as their body is effectively managing immune and inflammatory levels. Regardless, this discovery is promising and puts dexamethasone in the spotlight as a potentially life-saving intervention in critically ill COVID-19 patients.

The combination of its availability, its price, and its efficacy makes dexamethasone a breakthrough in coronavirus treatment plans, provided it continues to show results (myoclinic.com, 2020).

Mechanism of action of dexamethasone: Dexamethasone reduces inflammation by mimicking anti-inflammatory hormones produced by the body. Coronavirus infection triggers inflammation as the body tries to fight it off, and dexamethasone counter-acts it. According to a meta-analysis that aggregated seven randomized trials, Dexamethasone reduced mortality in critically ill patients with COVID-19 as well as in hospitalized patients with COVID-19 who required oxygen, particularly those receiving mechanical ventilation.

5. Interferons for treatment for COVID-19 sickness: Interferons are a family of cytokines with in vitro and in vivo antiviral properties.

Cytokines are proteins produced by cells, and they serve as molecular messengers between cells. In arthritis, cytokines regulate various inflammatory responses. As part of the immune system, cytokines regulate the body's response to disease and infection, as well as mediate normal cellular processes in your body. Interferon beta-1a has been approved by the Food and Drug Administration (FDA) to treat relapsing forms of multiple sclerosis, and it has been evaluated in clinical trials for the treatment of COVID-19. Interferon Alfa has been approved to treat hepatitis B and hepatitis C virus infections, and interferon lambda is not currently approved by the FDA for any use. Both interferon alfa and lambda have also been evaluated for the treatment of COVID-19 (www. verywellhealth.com., 2021).

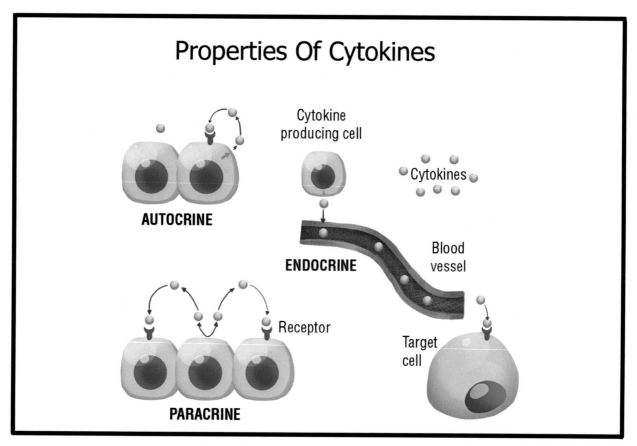

Fig. 4. Cytokines are immune modulating agents involved in autocrine, paracrine, and endocrine signaling (www.verywellhealth.com**., 2021).**

Cytokine is an umbrella term that includes many types of protein messengers, more specific names are given to cytokines based on either the type of cell that makes them or the action they have in the body. There are certainly over 100 separate genes coding for cytokine-like activities, many with overlapping functions and many still unexplored.

The definition of a cytokine is that it is as a soluble factor produced by one cell and acting on another cell, in order to bring about a change in the function of the target cell. In a way, one can consider cytokines as the "hormones" of immune and inflammatory responses. However, there are several properties of cytokines that escape this definition. For example, hormones are the primary product of a specific tissue or cell whereas cytokines are products of most cells. Most importantly, on a molar basis, cytokines are far more potent than hormones. For example, the concentration of the cytokine IL-1 that induces gene expression and synthesis of cyclo-oxygenase-1 (COX-2) is 10 pM and the ability of IL-12 to induce IFNγ is 20 pM. In fact, during purification of several cytokines from cell cultures, it was not uncommon to have a biological response in the absence of a visible band on gel electrophoresis. (C. A. Dinarello, 2007)

Cytokines are a broad and loose category of small proteins important in cell signaling, as described below:

Lymphokines are produced by lymphocytes (T cells) of the immune system. Lymphokines act to attract additional immune cells to mount an immune response, for instance in stimulating B cells to generate antibodies against the invading pathogen.

Monokines are produced primarily by monocytes and macrophages. Monokines include interleukin-1, tumor necrosis factor (TNF), α and β interferons and colony-stimulating factors. Monokines have regulatory effects on the functions of other cells, such as lymphocytes. The family of TNF includes over 20 members, each a separate gene product but with a considerable overlap in biological properties.

Chemokines send messages to other cells through a process called chemotaxis. There are two structural classes, the CC chemokines and the CXC chemokines. The messengers initiate the immune response by alerting other cells of threats and guiding them to the site of injury or infection. Interferons are proteins secreted in response to bacteria, viruses, parasites, or cancer cells. They inhibit virus replication by immediately signaling nearby cells to shield themselves from the virus and activating natural killer T-cells to destroy infected cells.

Interleukins (ILs) mediate communications between cells. Interleukins regulate cell growth, differentiation, and motility. Specific interleukins can have a major impact on cell-cell communication. So far 33 interleukins (genes and proteins) have been described.

Cytokines wreak havoc with the immune system turning against itself in autoimmune diseases. During infection, the cytokine "storm" subsides as the infection is eliminated and the genes return to their normal state of being repressed by histone acetylases. When cytokines genes fail to shut down, their products drive the host into a state of chronically activated cells, which now dominate an otherwise resting immune system. Auto-reactive T-cells are cells that persist and fail to die. There are likely other mechanisms of "failure to die" that account for the persistence which are influenced genetically. Most anti-cytokine therapies for autoimmune disease target the effects of cytokines on inflammatory and tissue remodeling processes but seem unable to shut down the persistently activated auto-reactive T-cell.

Cytokine storm has received more attention because of the COVID-19 pandemic. Cytokine storm syndrome refers to a group of related medical conditions in which the immune system is producing too many inflammatory signals, sometimes leading to organ failure and death (Hickman RJ 2021).

There are no specific drugs available to combat SARS-CoV-2 infection. Natural products (carolacton, homoharringtonine, emetine, and cepharanthine) are potential anti-SARS-CoV-2 agents that have attracted significant attention due to their broad-spectrum antiviral activities. Natural products possess tremendous structural diversity and unique chemical diversity, and they continue to serve as excellent starting points for inspiring new drug discovery. Growing understanding of efficient antiviral drug development has led to the exploration of natural products as an important tactic for identifying effective COVID-19 treatments.

Waiting in the Wings: *Antiviral drugs for COVID-19 are on the horizon at the urgency level. While a number of vaccines are available worldwide to prevent infection, there are limited treatment options for people infected with COVID-19.*

References:

——.2021. "Antiviral in the works." https://ateapharma.com/at-527/.

——. 2021. "Investigational oral antiviral." Ridgeback Biotherapeutics. Miami, FL, USA. www.ridgeback.biotherapeutics.com.

——. 2021. "Global access to drugs." Pfizer Pharmaceutical Company, New York City, NY, USA https://www.pfizer.com/.

——.2021. "Lavgevrio pill." Merck & Co, NJ, USA. www.Merck.com.

——. "Molnupiravir/ EIDD-2801." Merck & Co Inc/Handout/Reuters. Accessed Nov. 7, 2021.

——. 2021. "Remdesivir." Gilead Sciences, Inc., Foster City, CA 94404; www.gilead.com.

——. 2020. "Top Dexamethasone Manufacturers in the USA and Globally." www.marketwatch.com, https://www.thomasnet.com.

Albani, F., Fusina, F., Granato, E., et al. 2021, "Corticosteroid treatment has no effect on hospital mortality in COVID-19 patients." *Sci. Rep* 11: 1015. https://doi.org/10.1038/s41598-020-80654-x.

Auwaerter, P. G., Casadevall, A., Bloch, E. M., et al. 2021. "Deployment of convalescent plasma for the prevention and treatment of COVID-19." J Clin Invest. 130(6):2757-2765. doi:10.1172/JCI138745.

Buchy, P., Buisson, Y., Cintra, O., et al. 2021. "COVID-19 pandemic: lessons learned from more than a century of pandemics and current vaccine development for pandemic control" [published online ahead of print, 2021 Sep 23]. *Int J Infect Dis*.112:300-317. doi:10.1016/j.ijid.2021.09.045.

CEPI (Coalition for Epidemic Preparedness Innovations). "How COVAX will work. 2020b," accessed October 2020. https://cepi.net/COVAX/.

CIDRAP. 2020. "Universal influenza vaccine technology landscape," accessed on October 2020. https://www.cidrap.umn.edu/universal-influenzavaccine-technology-landscape.

Cortisone. 2021. Accessed on November 7. https://pubchem.ncbi.nlm.nih.gov/compound/Cortisone.

Dinarello, C. A. 2007. "Historical insights into cytokines." *Eur J Immunol 37 Suppl*: S34–45. Doi:10.1002/eji.200737772.

Glesby, M. J., Gulick, R. M., 2021. "Selecting treatments during an infectious disease pandemic: chasing the evidence." *Ann Intern Med*. 174(10): 1464-1465. doi:10.7326/M21-3221

Hickman, R. J. 2021. "What is cytokine storm syndrome? An exaggerated and dangerous immune response" https://www.h-h-c.com, updated Nov 04, 2021.

Lee, A., Blair, H. A. 2020. "Dexamethasone Intracanalicular Insert: A Review in Treating Post-Surgical Ocular Pain and Inflammation." *Drugs*, *80*(11), 1101–1108. https://doi.org/10.1007/s40265-020-01344-6.

Malin, J. J., Suarez, I., Priesner, V., et al. 2020. "Remdesivir against COVID-19 and Other Viral Diseases." *Clin Microbiol Rev.* 34(1): e00162-20. doi: 10.1128/CMR.00162-20.

Moscicki, R., 2021. "The important role of antivirals in the fight against COVID-19." https://catalyst.phrma.org/.

Pinzón, M. A., Ortiz, S., Holguín, H., et al. 2021. "Dexamethasone vs methylprednisolone high dose for Covid-19 pneumonia." *PLoS ONE* 16(5): e0252057. https://doi.org/10.1371/journal.pone.0252057.

Recovery Collaborative Group. 2021. "Therapeutic Management of Hospitalized Adults with COVID-19." *N Engl J Med 2021*, 384:693-704DOI: 10.1056/NEJMoa2021436.

Rhen, T., Cidlowski, J. A. 2005. "Anti-inflammatory action of glucocorticoids—new mechanisms for old drugs." *N Engl J Med.* 353(16):1711–23.

Sheahan, T. P., Frieman, M. B. 2020. "The continued epidemic threat of SARS-CoV-2 and implications for the future of global public health." *Curr Opin Virol*. doi: 10.1016/j.coviro.2020.05.010.

Study (Media/CNBC, Squawk on the Street, 10.01.2021).

Wahl, A., Gralinski, L. E., Johnson, C. E., et al. 2021. "SARS-CoV-2 infection is effectively treated and prevented by EIDD-2801." *Nature* 591(7850):451–457.

Willyard, C. 2021. "How antiviral pill molnupiravir shot ahead in the COVID drug hunt." *Nature*. doi: 10.1038/d41586-021-02783-1.

Wang, Z., Yang, L. 2020. "Turning the Tide: Natural Products and Natural-Product-Inspired Chemicals as Potential Counters to SARS-CoV-2 Infection." *Front Pharmacol*. 2020; 11:1013.

Image credit 2021, accessed Nov. 7, 2021, Joshimerbin/ Shutterstock.com.

Image credit: Joshimerbin/Shutterstock.com

www.marketwatch.com, 2020

https://www.thomasnet.com, 2020

www.ridgebackbiotherapeutics.com.

CHAPTER 7

SPIKE PROTEINS OF SARS-COV-2

The genome of SARS-CoV-2 encodes 29 viral proteins, including 16 nonstructural proteins (NSP1 to NSP16), 4 structural proteins, including spike (S), membrane (M), nucleocapsid (N), and envelope (E) proteins, and 9 accessory proteins.

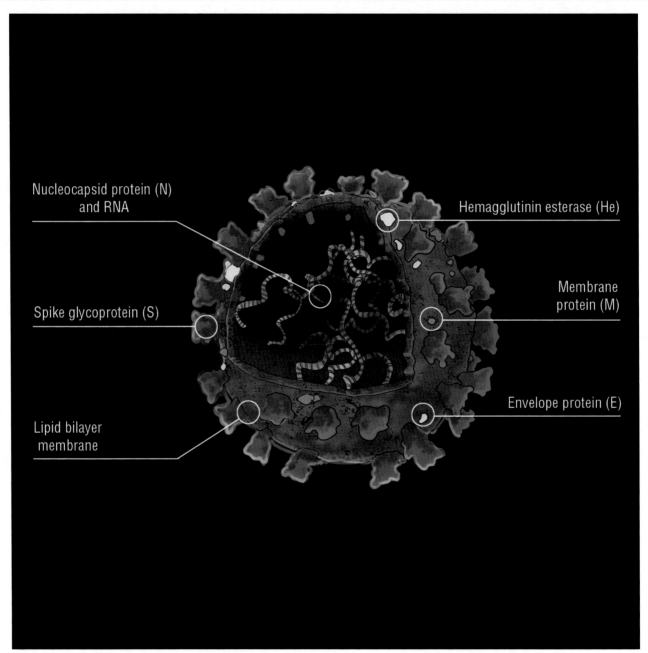

Fig. 1. Structure of COVID-19 virus (image credit: Orpheus FX/shutterstock.com).

The S proteins play a crucial role in penetrating host cells and initiating infection, whereas the M and E proteins are primarily involved in virus assembly.

Structure of spike proteins: The S proteins are large; an average CoV S protein contains 1,300 amino acids and 20 asparagine-linked glycans.

Glycan structures are modified monosaccharides, like N-Acetylglucosamine GlcNAc), N-Acetylgalactosamine (NGalNAc), or Sialic acid (N-Acetylneuraminic acid) (Neu5Ac). Glycotechnology is a developing field which is especially used in drug development.

The S protein monomers are assembled into trimers within the Endoplasmic reticulum of virus-producing cells and incorporated into virus particles at the CoV budding sites, at or near the ER-Golgi Intermediate Compartment.

The S protein is a highly glycosylated and large type I transmembrane fusion protein that is made up of 1,160 to 1,400 amino acids, depending upon the type of virus.

The presence of S proteins on the coronaviruses is what gives rise to the spike-shaped protrusions found on their surface.

S proteins of coronaviruses can be divided into two subunits:

The N-terminal S1 subunit—globular head of the S protein, the receptor-binding region.

The C-terminal S2 subunit—stalk of the protein, it is directly embedded into the viral envelope. It contains fusion peptide (FP), heptad repeats (HR1 and HR2), and transmembrane domain (TM). Arrows indicate the cleavage sites (fig. 2).

Spike proteins are assembled into trimers on the virion surface to form the distinctive corona or crown-like appearance.

Function of spike proteins: Upon interaction with a potential host cell, the S1 subunit will recognize and bind to receptors on the host cell, whereas the S2 subunit, which is the most conserved component of the S protein, will be responsible for fusing the envelope of the virus with the host cell membrane.

Once the S1 subunit binds to host cell receptors, two major conformational changes must occur for the S2 subunit to complete the fusion of the virus to the cell membrane. The two components of the S2 subunit that are involved in the coronavirus fusion include heptad repeat (HR) regions; HR1 and HR2.

The first conformation otherwise referred to as pre-hairpin, involves the transformation of an unstructured linker within the S2 subunit to become helical. The second conformational change to occur involves the inversion of this subunit's C-helix to the coil, resulting in the formation of a six-helix bundle.

Once these conformations are completed, the fusion peptide is anchored to the membrane of the host cell to allow the virus to move closer towards the cell membrane and eventually deliver the nucleo-capsid to the target cell.

Spike proteins induce neutralizing antibodies (NAbs) of the host cells: Nabs are protective antibodies that naturally produced by our humoral immune system. For example, 80R, CR3014, and CR3022, are some of the Nabs identified which specifically target the S1 domain of spike proteins of SARS-CoV induce T-cell responses and protective immunity.

People who had mild and brief COVID-19 infection, their immune system produced Nabs and neutralized the SARS-CoV-2.

People who recovered from mild COVID-19 infections produced antibodies circulating in their blood. The antibodies are the effective neutralizing immune response to the spike proteins.

A portion of this spiky surface appendage allows the virus to bind a receptor on human cells, causing other portions of the spike to fuse the viral and human cell membranes. This process is needed for the virus to gain entry into cells and infect them.

The convalescent plasma response to SARS-CoV-2 is oligo-clonal and directed overwhelmingly toward non-receptor binding domain (RBD) epitopes in the spike S1-ectodomain. The convalescent plasma response includes public and potently neutralizing antibodies (Nabs) against S1 spike protein. The mutations present in circulating SARS-CoV-2 variants can impair or ablate binding and neutralization by public N-terminal domain (NTD) of S1 spike protein may constitute a mechanism of viral escape in a subset of the population.

Antibodies to SARS-CoV-2 can target many of its encoded proteins, including structural and non-structural antigens.

The development of antibody is a common immunological phenomenon constantly happening in our body to give us protection, particularly against the newly invaded immunogens. In the case of COVID-19 infection, the antibody can be detected as soon as the first week from the onset of the symptoms depending on the patients' immune system. Several studies are ongoing around the world to track down the durability of anti-SARS-CoV-2 IgG (H. R. Choudhary et al. 2021).

The spike (S1) glycoproteins of coronaviruses bind to certain receptors on the host cells.

S1 binds to host receptors; Angiotensin-converting enzyme 2 (ACE2), Dipeptidyl peptidase-4 (DPP4), Aminopeptidase N (APN,), Carcino-embryonic antigen-related cell adhesion molecule-1(CEACAM,) and O-acetylated sialic acid (O-acetyl-Sia).

The term 'peplomer' is typically used to a grouping of heterologous proteins on the virus surface that function together. The spike (S) glycoprotein of coronaviruses is known to be essential in the binding of the virus to the host cell at the advent of the infection.

S2 contains basic elements needed for the SARS-CoV-2 to infect the human respiratory epithelial cells through interaction with the human ACE2 receptor. S1 mainly contains a receptor binding domain (RBD), which is responsible for recognizing the cell surface membrane fusion.

Though the primary target tissues of SARS-CoV-2 are airways and lungs, there is also evidence of direct viral infection of endothelial cells and diffuse endothelial inflammation in COVID-19 disease. Moreover, vulnerable patients with pre-existing endothelial dysfunction, which is associated with male sex, smoking, hypertension, diabetes, obesity, and established cardiovascular disease, are associated with adverse outcomes in COVID-19.

The viral infection of endothelial cells plays a central role in the pathogenesis of Acute Respiratory Distress Syndrome (ARDS) and multi-organ failure in patients with COVID-19. Therefore, the vascular system is increasingly being addressed as a major therapeutic target for defeating COVID-19. COVID-19's wide variety of seemingly unconnected complications, and could open the door for new research into more effective therapies.

The S1 of SARS-CoV-2 induces blood platelets: SARS-CoV-2-induced platelet activation causes thrombus formation and inflammatory responses in COVID-19 patients. Platelet activation is critical for thrombosis and is responsible for the thrombotic events and cardiovascular complications.

Transmembrane protease spliced serine 2 (TMPRSS2) of the host plays a critical role in the binding of S1 to ACE2 receptor cell entry in synergetic manner. The viral S glycoprotein is cleaved by TMPRSS2, thus facilitating viral activation and representing one of the essential host factors for SARS-CoV-2 pathogenicity. The ACE-bound spike of the virus is cleaved (activated) by TMPRSS2 protease which allows the virus to enter into the human cell surface membrane either by endocytosis or fusion with the surface membrane.

This process is similar to viral activation and cell entry of other coronaviruses, including SARS-CoV, as well as influenza virus such as influenza H1N1.

Since COVID-19 is a disease previously unknown to human beings, no proven treatments exist at present and the most important public health solution would be an effective vaccine.

Spike protein deletions and mutations linked to COVID-19 surges. The surges in COVID-19 case numbers have been associated with deletions and mutations in the SARS-CoV-2 genome in an antigenic site of the spike proteins. The N-terminal domain (NTD) of the virus's spike protein (S1) has appeared as a potentially mutable structure that may allow the virus to escape antibody neutralization.

The deletions and mutations in virus assist in evading immunity and potentially play a role in surges infections" (A. Manjarrez, 2021).

It is hard to tell whether the mutations came first or the surges came first. When lots of people got sick all over the world, and also virus replicated, which lead to more viral mutations. So both things happened simultaneously. The surge is not dependent just on the virus, but also on many other factors; mutations in the virus, susceptibility to different hosts, human and other animals, and protection measures (T. Hatziioannou, 2021).

Spike proteins cause mitochondrial fragmentation in the cells:

"The binding of spike proteins disrupted ACE2's molecular signaling to mitochondria (organelles that generate energy for cells), causing the mitochondria to become damaged and fragmented.

"Confocal images of vascular endothelial cells treated with Spike S1 protein revealed increased mitochondrial fragmentation, indicating altered mitochondrial dynamics" **(Y. Lei et al. 2021)**

Spike proteins (S1 and S2) mediated the fusion process for entry of SARS-CoV-2 into the human cells: The spike S1 plays a key role in the early steps of viral infection in binding to the receptor, and the S2 protein mediates membrane fusion.

"Among all structural proteins of SARS-CoV, spike protein is the main antigenic component that is responsible for inducing host immune responses, neutralizing antibodies and/or protective immunity against virus infection. Spike protein has therefore been selected as an important target for coronavirus vaccine and anti-viral development" (S. Belouzard et al. 2009).

"CoV diversity is reflected in the variable S proteins, which have evolved into forms differing in their receptor interactions and their response to various environmental triggers of virus-cell membrane fusion. As such, seemingly minor differences in CoV S protein structure and function often correlate with striking changes in CoV tropism and virulence.

"The main functions for the Spike protein are summarized as: Mediate receptor binding and membrane fusion; Defines the range of the hosts and specificity of the virus; Main component to bind with the neutralizing antibody; Key target for vaccine design; Can be transmitted between different hosts through gene recombination or mutation of the receptor binding domain (RBD), leading to a higher mortality rate" (www.mdpi.com, accessed on Nov. 11, 2021).

As we have noted, there are still significant gaps in our knowledge of the virus-receptor interactions and the S protein triggering to catalyze the membrane fusion of the human cell with the SARS-CoV-2. New articles show up to our surprise to bridge or address the gaps. It is a good model system of virus-receptor interactions and is bringing out new insights into the relevance of viruses in general.

References:

Belouzard, S., Chu, V. C., Whittaker, G. R. 2009. "Activation of the SARS coronavirus spike protein via sequential proteolytic cleavage at two distinct sites." *PNAS* 106(14): 5875.

Belouzard, S., Millet, J. K., Licitra, B. N., et al. 2012. "Mechanisms of Coronacirus Cell Entry Mediated by the Viral Spike Protein." *Viruses* 4(6):1011-1033. doi:10.3390/v4061011.

Choudhary, H. R., Parai, D., Dash, G. C., et al. 2021. "IgG antibody response against nucleocapsid and spike protein post-SARS-CoV-2 infection." *Infection* 49(5):1045-1048. doi: 10.1007/s15010-021-01651-4. Epub 2021 Jul 2. PMID: 34213733; PMCID: PMC8249824.

Hatziioannou, T. 2021. "Research Program on COVID-19/SARS-COV-2," accessed Nov. 12, 2021. www.rockefeller.edu/.

Lei, Y., Zhang, J., Schiavon, C. R. 2021. "SARS-CoV-2 Spike protein impairs endothelial function via downregulation of ACE 2." *Circ Res.* 128(9):1323–1326. doi:10.1161/CIRCRESAHA.121.318902.

Manjarrez, A. 2021. "Spike protein deletions linked to COVID-19 surges." https://www.the-scientistcom.

Mollica, V., Rizzo, A., Massari, F. 2020. "The pivotal role of TMPRSS2 in coronavirus disease 2019 and prostate cancer."

Future Oncology. 16(27):2029–2033.

Montopoli, M., Zumerle, S., Vettor, R., et al. 2020. "Androgen-deprivation therapies for prostate cancer and risk of infection by SARS-CoV-2: a population-based study (n=4532)." *Ann Oncol.* 31(8): 1040–1045. doi: 10.1016/j.annonc.2020.04.479.

Qian, Y., Lei, T., Patel, P. S., et al. 2021. "Direct activation of endothelial cells by SARS-CoV-2 nucleocapsid protein is blocked by Simvastatin." *J Virol* 95(23): e0139621. doi: 10.1128/ JVI.01396-21.

Voss, W. N., Hou, Y. J., Johnson NV, et al. 2021. "Prevalent protective and convergent IgG recognition of SARS-CoV-2 non-RBD spike epitopes." *Science.* 372 (6546): 1108–1112. doi: 10.1126/science.abg5268. PMID: 33947773.

Zhang, S., Liu, Y., Wang, X., et al. 2020. "SARS-CoV-2 binds platelet ACE2 to enhance thrombosis in COVID-19." *J Hematol Oncol.* 13(1):120. Published Sept. 4, 2020. doi:10.1186/ s13045-020-00954-7.

htpps://www.mdpi.com, accessed, Nov. 11, 2021.

CHAPTER 8

M PROTEINS OF SARS-COV-2

The M protein of coronavirus plays a central role in virus assembly, turning cellular membranes into workshops where virus and host factors come together to make new virus particles.

Using the techniques of cryo-electron microscopy, tomography, and statistical analysis, it was shown that M proteins adopt two conformations.

> 1. Elongated M protein is associated with rigidity, clusters of spikes, and a relatively narrow range of membrane curvature.

> 2. In contrast, compact M protein is associated with flexibility and low spike density.

"Analysis of several types of virus-like particles and virions revealed that S protein, N protein and genomic RNA each help to regulate virion size and variation, presumably through interactions with M. These findings provide insight into how M protein functions to promote virus assembly particles" (B. W. Neuman et al. 2011).

As we mentioned earlier, the viral particle is composed of 4 structural proteins. spike (S), envelope (E), membrane (M), and nucleoprotein (N). The involvement of each of these proteins, and their interactions are critical for the assembly and production of coronavirus particles.

Using *in silico* analyses, the structure, and potential function of the M protein were determined. An *in silico* experiment is one performed on a computer or via computer simulation. The phrase is pseudo-Latin for in silicon and refers to silicon in computer chips.

In silico analyses showed that the M protein of SARS-CoV-2 has a triple helix bundle, forms a single 3-trans-membrane domain, and is homologous to the prokaryotic sugar transport protein SemiSWEET. SemiSWEETs are related to the PQ-loop family whose members function as cargo receptors in vesicle transport, mediate movement of basic amino acids across lysosomal membranes, and are also involved in phospholipase flippase function (fig. 1).

"Eukaryotic SWEETs are composed of 7 transmembrane helices (TMHs) that contain a pair of 3 transmembrane repeats, which are connected by an additional helix. SWEETs in prokaryotes, contain 3 TMHs. The human genome contains only 1 *SWEET* gene and may be involved in glucose transport" (L. Q. Chen et al. 2010).

The SWEET (sugars will eventually be exported transporter) family, also known as the PQ-loop. PQ-loop proteins possess two well-conserved repeat sequences termed PQ-loop motif, the Proline-Glutamine dipeptide.

The sugar transporter-like structure of M protein influences glycosylation of the S protein.

Endocytosis is critical for the internalization and maturation of RNA viruses, including SARS-CoV-2. Overall, the semi-SWEET sugar transporter structure of the M protein is involved in multiple functions that may aid in the rapid proliferation, replication, and immune evasion of the SARS-CoV-2 virus.

M protein is the most abundant structural protein of coronaviruses that spans the membrane bilayer and binds to all other structural proteins and stabilizes the complex inside the virion. Engineering of SWEET mutants using genomic editing tools has been shown to mediate resistance to pathogens. (S. Thomas, 2020).

Structure of M proteins of SARS-CoV-2: "Three-dimensional (3D) structures of proteins provide valuable insights into their function on a molecular level and a broad spectrum of applications in life science research. A detailed description of the interactions of proteins and the overall quaternary structure is essential for a comprehensive understanding of biological systems, how protein complexes and networks operate, and how they could be modulated. SWISS-MODEL is a server that is used for

3-D structure prediction. SWISS-MODEL is the first fully automated protein homology modeling server and is updated continuously. Its functionality has been extended to the modeling of homo- and hetero-meric complexes. Starting from the amino acid sequences of the interacting proteins, both the stoichiometry and the overall structure of the complex are inferred by homology modelling. The SWISS-MODEL (expasy.org) has modelled the full SARS-CoV-2 proteome based on the NCBI reference sequence NC_045512 and annotations from UniProt.

The complete nucleic acid sequence of NC_045512 has been determined.

"NC_045512; single stranded RNA (ss-RNA) of SARS-CoV-2; has 29903 bases" ("Severe acute respiratory syndrome coronavirus 2 isolate Wuhan-Hu-1, co - Nucleotide – NCBI", nih.gov).

Here is the summary of the sequence:
ORIGIN

```
  1 attaaaggtt tataccttcc caggtaacaa accaaccaac tttcgatctc ttgtagatct
 61 gttctctaaa cgaactttaa aatctgtgtg gctgtcactc ggctgcatgc ttagtgcact
121 cacgcagtat aattaataac taattactgt cgttgacagg acacgagtaa ctcgtctatc
181 ttctgcaggc tgcttacggt ttcgtccgtg ttgcagccga tcatcagcac atctaggttt
241 cgtccgggtg tgaccgaaag gtaagatgga gagccttgtc cctggtttca acgagaaaac
```

```
29701 gggaggactt gaaagagcca ccacattttc accgaggcca cgcggagtac gatcgagtgt
```

29761 acagtgaaca atgctaggga gagctgccta tatggaagag ccctaatgtg
taaaattaat

29821 tttagtagtg ctatccccat gtgattttaa tagcttctta ggagaatgac
aaaaaaaaaa

29881 aaaaaaaaaa aaaaaaaaaa aaa

//

Fig. 1. Sequence of single-stranded RNA of SARS-CoV-2 gene (29903
bases) (NC-045512) (ncbi-nih.gov, accessed 2021).

The structural protein sequence in the single amino acid code of the M
protein of SARS-CoV-2 is shown in fig. 3.

QJA17755.1 membrane glycoprotein
[Severe acute respiratory syndrome coronavirus 2]

1 madsngtitv eelkklleqw nlvigflflt wicllqfaya nrnrflyiik liflwllwpv
61 tlacfvlaav yrinwitggi aiamaclvgl mwlsyfiasf rlfartrsmw sfnpetnill
121 nvplhgtilt rplleselvi gavilrghlr iaghhlgrcd ikdlpkeitv atsrtlsyyk
181 lgasqrvagd sgfaaysryr ignyklntdh ssssdniall vq

Fig. 2. Amino acid sequence of membrane glycoprotein of SARS-
CoV-2 (QJA17755.1) (ncbi-nih.gov, accessed 2021).

As shown in fig. 2, there are a total of 222 amino acids in M glycoprotein of
SARS-CoV-2 starting with m (methionine) and ending with Q (glutamine).

The Single Letter Amino acid Code:

G	Glycine	Gly		**P**	Proline	Pro
A	Alanine	Ala		**V**	Valine	Val
L	Leucine	Leu		**I**	Isoleucine	Ile
M	Methionine	Met		**C**	Cysteine	Cys
F	Phenylalanine	Phe		**Y**	Tyrosine	Tyr
W	Tryptophan	Trp		**H**	Histidine	His
K	Lysine	Lys		**R**	Arginine	Arg
Q	Glutamine	Gln		**N**	Asparagine	Asn
E	Glutamic Acid	Glu		**D**	Aspartic Acid	Asp
S	Serine	Ser		**T**	Threonine	Thr

Fig. 3. Amino acid sequence code (ncbi-nih.gov, accessed 2021).

The amino acid sequence of the M protein was entered into the SWISS-MODEL server and I-TASSER. Based on the sequence, the structure of the molecule was predicted as the bidirectional sugar transporter.

The transmembrane structure of SARS-CoV-2 membrane M is shown in fig. 4.

SARS-CoV-2 membrane protein (M)

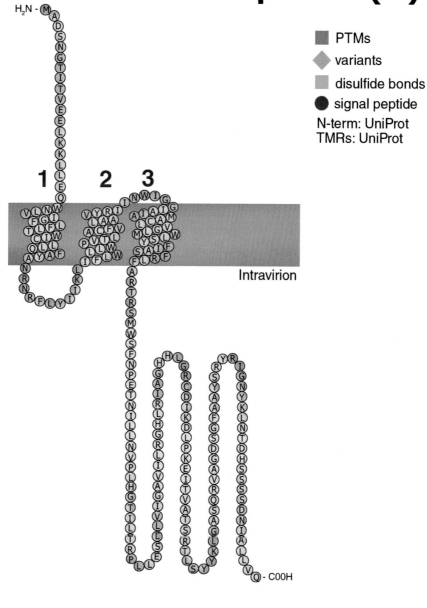

Fig. 4. Transmembrane structure of SARS-CoV-2 membrane M (*PubMed Central*, 2020).

Membrane topology of proteins (snake diagrams) determined using Protter.

The membrane (M) glycoprotein of SARS-CoV-2 has a triple helix bundle and formed a single 3-transmembrane domain.

ClustalW2 was used to determine homology between M proteins of different coronaviruses. SARS-CoV-2 M protein has a sequence similarity of 98.6% with the M protein of bat SARS-CoV, 98.2% homology with the pangolin SARS-CoV, 89.14% similarity with the M protein of SARS-CoV and a sequence similarity of 38.36% with the M protein of MERS-CoV.

In vitro studies show that all structural proteins are required for the production of SARS-CoV-2: Coexpression of all structural proteins, S, E, M, and N, was the most efficient combination to induce virus-like particle VLP secretion in the mammalian expression system.

"Virus-like particles are molecules that closely resemble viruses, but are non-infectious because they do not contain viral genetic material. Virus-like particles are also very small, with a particle radius of approximately 20 to 200 nm. Virus-Like Particles (VLPs) and Nano-Particles (NPs) are being used for vaccine development They are very effective way of creating vaccines against deadly viruses, such as SARS-CoV-2, human papilloma virus (HPV), hepatitis B, malaria, and more" (Perotti and Perez, 2019).

References:

Chen, L. Q., Hou, B. H., Lalonde, S., et al. 2010. "Sugar transporters for intercellular exchange and nutrition of pathogens.} *Nature*:

468; 527-532. DOI: 10.1038/nature09606.

Deng, D., Yan, N. 2016. "GLUT, SGLT, and SWEET: Structural and mechanistic investigations of the glucose transporters." *Protein Sci.* 25: 546–558. DOI: 10.1002/pro.2858.

Neuman, B. W., Kiss, G., Kunding, A. H., et al. 2011. "A structural analysis of M protein in coronavirus assembly and morphology." *J Struct Biol* 174:11–22.

Perotti, M., Perez, L. 2019. "Virus-Like Particles and Nanoparticles for vaccine development against HCMV." *Viruses.* 12(1):35. doi: 10.3390/v12010035.

Pubmed Central. 2020. *Pathog Immun* 5(1): 342-363.doi; 10.20411/pai.v5i1.377. nih.gov.

Thomas, S. 2020. "The Structure of the Membrane Protein of SARS-CoV-2 Resembles the Sugar Transporter SemiSWEET." *Pathog Immun.* 5(1):342-363. doi: 10.20411/pai.v5i1.377. PMID: 33154981; PMCID: PMC7608487.

Xu, R., Shi, M., Li, J., Song, P., Li, N. 2020. "Construction of SARS-CoV-2 Virus-Like Particles by Mammalian Expression System." *Front Bioeng Biotechnol.* 8:862. doi: 10.3389/fbioe.2020.00862. PMID: 32850726; PMCID: PMC7409377.

CHAPTER 9

ENVELOPE (E) PROTEINS OF SARS-COV-2

The SARS-CoV-2 envelope (E) protein (~8-12 kDa) is the smallest of the major structural proteins; Envelope (E), Membrane (M), Nucleoprotein (N), and Spike (S).

E protein is involved in many aspects of the viral life cycle, such as assembly, budding, envelope formation, and pathogenesis. It functions as an anion-channelling viroporin, and interacts with other CoV proteins and host cell proteins. Viroporins are a diverse class of small, hydrophobic virus-encoded membranes.

The deletion of E protein weakens or even abolishes the virulence of SARS-CoV-2.

Structure of SARS-CoV-2 envelope (E) protein: The E forms an ion-channel termed as viroporin. Viroporins are expressed by a diverse set of viruses and have been found to target nearly every host cell membrane and compartment, including endocytic/exocytic vesicles, endoplasmic reticulum, mitochondria, Golgi, and the plasma membrane. Viroporins are generally very small (<100 amino acids) integral membrane proteins that share common structure motifs (conserved cluster of basic residues adjacent to an amphipathic alpha-helix) but with only limited sequence homology between viruses. Ion channel activity of viroporins is either required for replication or it greatly enhances replication and pathogenesis (J. M. Hyser, 2015).

Structure of E protein of SARS-CoV-2: The diagrammic representation of the structure of E protein is shown in fig.1.

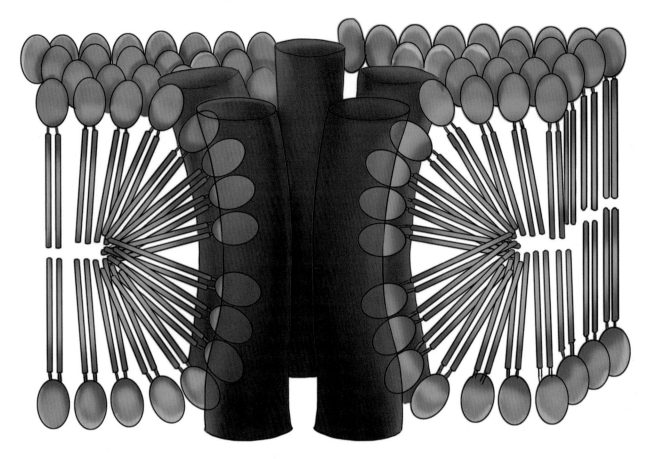

Fig.1. Structure of SARS-CoV E protein proteolipid ion channel (Y. Cao et al. 2021).

Phospholipids are represented in blue, and E protein monomers are shown as red cylinders. Lipid head groups (blue ellipses) also face the ion channel lumen.

"Viroporin channel currents range between highly variable ('burst-like') fluctuations to well resolved unitary ('square-top') transitions, and emerging data indicates that the quality of channel activity is influenced by many factors, including viroporin synthesis/solubilization, the lipid environment and the ionic composition of the buffers, as well as intrinsic differences between the viroporins themselves" (J. M. Hyser, 2015).

"Compounds that block viroporin channel activity are effective antiviral drugs both *in vitro* and *in vivo*. Surprisingly distinct viroporins are inhibited by the same compounds (e.g., amantadines and amiloride derivatives), despite wide sequence divergence, raising the possibility of broadly acting antiviral drugs that target viroporins

"Electrophysiology of viroporins plays a critical role in pathogenesis and this property of viroporins is being utilized to develop new drugs to combat viroporin-encoding pathogens" (J. M. Hyser, 2015).

"The selectivity of SARS-CoV E protein ion channel depends on the charge of the lipid membranes. The lipid head-groups are an integral component of the channel pore.

Several SARS-CoV-2 proteins, including E, ORF3a and ORF8a, can self-assemble into oligomers and generate ion channels (fig.2)" (Y. Cao et al. 2021).

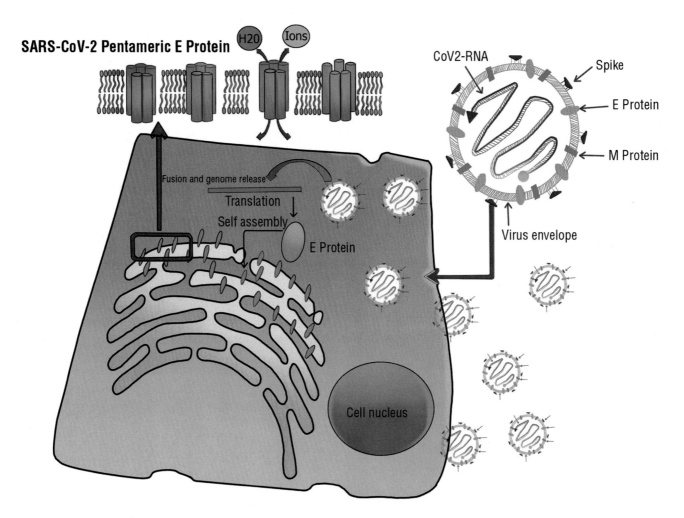

Fig. 2. E protein monomer self-assembles into an oligomer that functions as an ion channel (Y. Cao et al. 2021).

The lipid envelope encloses the virus and facilitates the entry of the SARS-coronavirus (CoV)-2 E protein into the host cell. The E protein is translated in the endoplasmic reticulum (ER) and accumulates in the Golgi. Then, the E protein monomer self-assembles into an oligomer that functions as an ion channel (fig.2).

The influence of SARS-CoV E protein ion channel activity in cell ion homeostasis is highly dependent on its subcellular localization. After SARS-CoV infection, E protein mainly accumulates in the Endoplasmic Reticulum Golgi Intermediate Compartment (ERGIC) region of the infected cells, where virus morphogenesis and budding take place. Ionic imbalances within cells can interfere with innate immunity and affect virus pathogenesis. Interestingly, disruption of ion gradients within the endoplasmic reticulum and Golgi apparatus by viral proteins with ion channel activity has been shown to delay protein transport preventing Major Histocompatibility Complex (MHC) molecules. The MHC molecules are the cell surface proteins essential for the adaptive immune system.

Mutations in E protein of SARS-CoV-2 result in attenuated viruses: "The introduction of point mutations that inhibited SARS-CoV E protein ion channel activity led to attenuated viruses, without significantly affecting virus production. Viruses displaying E protein ion channel activity caused an increased damage within pulmonary epithelia, which correlated with edema accumulation It has been shown that deletion of full-length E protein or modification of active motifs present in this protein have been essential to achieve two aims, the engineering of vaccine candidates that provide full-protection against homologous and heterologous CoVs, and the identification of drugs that interfere with exacerbated pathways responsible for disease severity. These drugs increase experimental animals' survival and, therefore, are good candidates as antivirals in human health" (Y. Cao et al. 2021).

Mutations generated by reverse genetics in E protein (M. L. DeDiego et al. 2014): "CoVs have evolved viral proteins that target different signaling pathways to counteract innate immune responses. A comprehensive accumulation of data has shown that the relatively small E protein elicits a strong influence on the interaction of SARS-CoV with the host. In fact, after infection with SARS-CoV-2 in which E protein has been deleted, increased cellular stress and unfolded protein responses, apoptosis, and augmented host immune responses were observed. In contrast, the presence of E protein activated a pathogenic inflammatory response that may cause death in animal models and in humans."

SARS-CoV E protein sequence and different virus mutants generated by reverse genetics are shown in fig. 3.

SARS-CoV-2 Nucleocapsid domain organization and interaction with the virus RNA

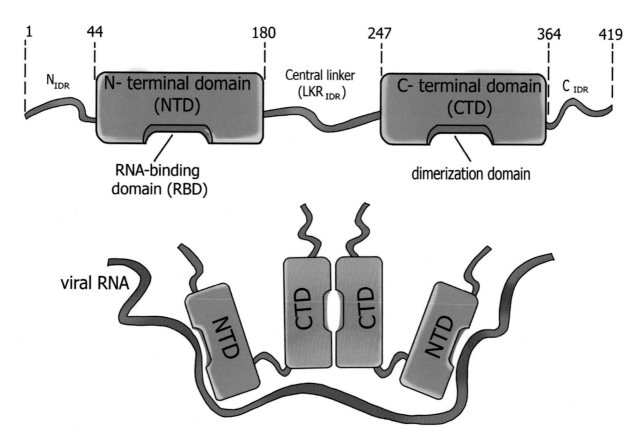

Fig. 3. Recombinant SARS-CoVs with E protein PBM truncated or mutated by reverse genetics (J. M. Jimenez-Guardeño et al. 2014).

The modification or deletion of different motifs within E protein, including the transmembrane domain that harbors an ion channel activity, small sequences within the middle region of the carboxy-terminus of E protein, and its most carboxy-terminal end, which contains a PDZ domain-binding motif (PBM), is sufficient to attenuate the virus.

(PBM stands for PDZ binding motif (PBM), and the PDZ is post-synaptic density zonulaoccludens-1).

As shown in fig. 3:

SARS-CoV-E-wt (wild type), C-terminal end has the sequence: DLLV, and the virulence level is +ve.
D is aspartic acid; L is leucine; L is leucine; V is valine.
SARS-CoV-E- deleted (delta) PBM, and the virulence level is −ve.
SARS-CoV-E-mutPBM, replacing DLLV with GGGG (where G is glycine), and the virulence level is −ve.
SARS-CoV-E-potPBM, replacing DLLV with ALAV (where A is Alanine), and the virulence level is +ve.

In SARS-CoV-E-potPBM, four amino acids of E protein were replaced by alanine, to generate a new potential PBM. Red boxes highlight PBMs within E protein. The gray box on the right indicates the virulence of the mutants: (+) indicates a virulent phenotype and (−) indicates an attenuated phenotype.

SARS-CoV E protein PBM is a molecular determinant of virulence. The recombinant viruses missing E protein PBM were generated. Infection of mice with the recombinant viruses lacking the E protein PBM led to a decrease in the deleterious, exacerbated immune response triggered during SARS-CoV infection and a lower expression of inflammatory cytokines, without significantly affecting virus titers in mice lungs. To understand the molecular basis of this attenuation, host factors interacting with E protein PBM were identified using proteomic studies. Specific interaction of this motif with the cellular protein syntenin, a relevant scaffolding protein that participates in the activation of p38 mitogen-activated protein kinase (MAPK), was found. Interestingly, activated p38 MAPK, which mediates the expression of proinflammatory cytokines was specifically reduced in mice infected with viruses missing E protein PBM, as compared with viruses containing this motif. These results highlight a novel mechanism of modulation of SARS-CoV pathogenesis by E protein. The interference with this signaling pathway will allow the development of therapies to reduce the exacerbated immune response triggered during SARS-CoV infection (J. M. Jimenez-Guardeno et al. 2014).

Bioinformatics analysis showed that other human CoV E proteins, such as that from MERS-CoV, HCoV-229E, HCoV-NL63, HCoV-OC43 and HCoV-HKU1 also encode a PBM in its carboxy-terminus. Therefore, the antiviral strategies described above to prevent SARS-CoV, most probably also apply to the reduction of the pathogenesis induced by other human CoVs. Furthermore, the generation of human attenuated coronaviruses by deleting E protein PBM could be the basis for the development of recombinant vaccines, as those described by deleting the whole SARS-CoV E protein or internal domains of this protein (M. L. DeDiego et al. 2014).

Effect of SARS-CoV E protein ion channel activity (EIC) in lung pathology: The lung histopathology in mice infected with a virus displaying (EIC$^+$) or lacking (EIC$^-$) E protein ion channel activity at four days post-infection (dpi) was conducted.

Evaluation of key inflammatory cytokines involved in epithelial damage and edema accumulation revealed that IL-1β, TNF and IL-6 amounts were increased in the lung airways of the mice infected with the viruses displaying E protein ion conductivity compared to the infection with the mutants lacking IC activity. IL-1β is one of the most important proinflammatory cytokines involved in Acute Respiratory Distress Syndrome (ARDS). IL-1β activation occurs when the inflammasome complex is stimulated by viral proteins with ion channel activity. Inflammatory response elicited by IL-1β is accompanied by an increase in TNF, and both signals are amplified by the accumulation of IL-6, which are key events during ARDS progression after SARS-CoV infection.

Studies on E gene deletion in SARS-CoV and its effects on viral pathogenesis: The E gene deletions in the virus were constructed and its effects on pathogenesis were studied. The lack of expression of E gene decreased its pathogenicity in Golden Syrian hamsters and in transgenic mice expressing the SARS-CoV receptor hACE-2. The rSARS-CoV-ΔE titers (the number of copies) decreased in vivo, in comparison to parental virus titers.

Function of SARS-CoV-2 envelope (E) protein: The biochemical and imaging assays were performed in infected versus transfected cells. It revealed that E protein along with the M protein regulate the intracellular trafficking of S as well as its intracellular processing. The imaging data reveals that S is relocalized at endoplasmic reticulum-golgi intermediate compartment (ERGIC) or Golgi compartments upon coexpression of E or M, as observed in SARS-CoV-2-infected cells, which prevents syncytia formation.

The C-terminal retrieval motif in the cytoplasmic tail of S is required for its M-mediated retention in the ERGIC, whereas E induces S retention by modulating the cell secretory pathway. The E and M induce a specific maturation of N-glycosylation of S, independently of the regulation of its localization, with a profile that is observed both in infected cells and in purified viral particles. The E, M, and N are required for the optimal production of virus-like particles.

The first functional evidence of SARS-CoV E protein acting as a viroporin was provided after its expression in bacteria, where E protein oligomerized and modified membrane permeability. Direct measurement of E protein ion channel activity was first reported using synthetic peptides representing full-length SARS-CoV E protein or its N-terminal 40 amino acids, including the transmembrane domain, in artificial lipid membranes. The E protein ion channel (EIC) activity was confirmed, and mutations that suppressed this function were identified. In addition, compounds that inhibit the SARS-CoV E protein ion conductivity were described, although their efficacy in the context of a viral infection was not reported.

SARS-CoV-2 E could modify the cell secretory pathway *via* a mechanism shared with some other coronaviruses. Previous reports indicated that the viroporins from divergent viruses can modulate the cell secretory pathway by different mechanisms. For example, the M2 protein from the influenza virus has a direct effect on late steps of plasma membrane delivery by delaying late Golgi transport, which indirectly affects the efficiency of earlier transport steps by altering the ionic content of the Golgi apparatus and the endosomes. Thus, it is plausible that the modulation of the cell secretory pathway by E could be important for the assembly of infectious particles by allowing the accumulation of the viral structural components at the virion assembly site. Alternatively, the modulation of the cell secretory pathway *per se* could be independent of virion assembly, but rather linked to virulence and/or induction of inflammasome since E was found to be associated to the virulence of several coronavirus genera, *e.g.*, for SARS-CoV or IBV as well as induction of the inflammasome for SARS-CoV.

Expression of SARS-CoV-2 E and M modulates the N-glycosylation pathway: E and M regulate the maturation of N glycosylation of S. E and M are located at the ERGIC and/or Golgi membranes. Although it was not possible to confirm this for SARS-CoV-2 E and M, owing to the unavailability of specific antibodies, it is likely that they share the ERGIC/Golgi intracellular localization. Since the maturation of N-glycans occurs in the Golgi, one possibility is that accumulation of E and M proteins at the membrane of this organelle could induce changes that alter the correct action of glycosyltransferases and hence, the N-glycan profile of SARS-CoV-2 S. While further studies would be required to determine the role of this modulation of S N-glycosylation maturation, one possibility is that this might modulate virion attachment to some lectins found at the cell surface. A recent study proposed that SARS-CoV S can bind different types of lectin and more particularly LSECtin, which can enhance infection in permissive cells. Accordingly, it is possible that, as shown in our report for SARS-CoV-2, the β-coronaviruses have developed mechanisms to control N-glycosylation pathway for their benefit.

Mutation of the gene encoding the E protein promotes apoptosis: E protein is embedded in the viral lipids that lead to the formation of SARS-CoV-2's inner core of Virus-like Particles, which promote the assembly of viruses and the mutations in it promote apoptosis.

E protein is expressed at a high level in each infected cell, but only a small amount of this expressed E protein is inserted into the viral membrane. Recombinant CoVs lacking the E protein show a significant reduction in viral titer and maturity or produce incompetent offspring.

Therapeutics to pathogenesis by E protein of SARS-CoV: One potential therapeutic approach is to target the pentameric E protein channels through viroporin inhibitors.

Hexamethylene amiloride and Amantadine and their combinations represent a broad range of viroporin inhibitors. These two compounds were obtained by screening 372 compounds in the MedChemExpress library and found that these were potential E protein channel inhibitors

E protein could be involved in multiple important aspects, from the assembly and induction of membrane curvature to division or budding and release to apoptosis, inflammation and even autophagy. The E protein is involved in many aspects of the viral replication cycle through the formation of oligomers and viroporins. The ion selectivity of the viroporin in the ER/Golgi membrane strongly affects the maintenance of the ion balance of the host cell microenvironment, pH and TMV. There are limited studies on the mechanism of the E protein viroporin in virus-infected cells according to the current understanding. Although in vitro experiments have shown that some inhibitors can effectively block the E protein viroporin of SARS-CoV-2 and weaken or abolish the virulence of the virus, their exact therapeutic effect remains to be further explored.

References:

Boston, R, Legros, V., Zhou, B. 2020. "The SARS-CoV-2 envelope and membrane proteins modulate maturation and retention of the spike protein, allowing assembly of virus-like particles." *J Biol Chem.* 296: 100111:1-13. https://doi.org/10.1074/jbc.RA120.016175.

Cao, Y., Yang, R., Lee, I., et al. 2021. "Characterization of the SARS-CoV-2 E Protein: Sequence, Structure, Viroporin, and Inhibitors." *Protein Sci.* 6:1114-1130. doi: 10.1002/pro.4075.

DeDiego, M. L., Nieto-Torres, J. L., Jimenez-Guardeno, J. M., et al. 2014. "Coronavirus virulence genes with main focus on SARS-CoV envelope gene." *Virus Res* 194:124-137. doi: 10.1016/j.virusres.2014.07.024.

Hyser, J. M. 2015. "Viroporins." *Electrophysiology of Unconventional Channels and Pores*.18:153–81. doi: 10.1007/978-3-319-20149-8_7.

Jimenez-Guardeño, J. M., Nieto-Torres, J. L., DeDiego, M. L., et al. 2014. "The PDZ-binding motif of severe acute respiratory syndrome coronavirus envelope protein is a determinant of viral pathogenesis." *PLoS Pathog.* 10(8): e1004320. doi: 10.1371/journal.ppat.1004320.

Nieto-Torres, J. L., DeDiego, M. L., Verdia-Baguena, C., et al. 2014. "Severe acute respiratory syndrome coronavirus envelope protein ion channel activity promotes virus fitness and pathogenesis." *PLoS Pathog.* 10(5): e1004077. doi: 10.1371/journal.ppat.1004077.

Teoh, K. T., Siu, Y. L., Chan, W. L.., et al. 2010. "The SARS coronavirus E protein interacts with PALS1 and alters tight junction formation and epithelial morphogenesis." *Mol Biol Cell* 21(22):3838-52. Doi:10.1091/mbc.E10-04-0338.

www.medchemexpress.com, accessed on February 16, 2022.

CHAPTER 10

N PROTEINS OF SARS-COV-2

The SARS-CoV nucleocapsid (N) protein is a structural protein that plays a primary role in packaging the viral genome into long, flexible, helical, complexes, and enhances the efficiency of viral transcription and assembly.

Structure of the SARS-CoV nucleocapsid (N) protein: Coronavirus assembly is mediated by specific interactions of the M protein with S, N, and E proteins.

The coronavirus nucleocapsid (N) is a structural protein that forms complexes with genomic RNA and interacts with the viral membrane protein during virion assembly. Recent studies have confirmed that N is a multifunctional protein.

N and M proteins are the two major structural proteins in CoV virions. The M protein is anchored by its three transmembrane domains to the viral envelope and its large carboxy-terminal tail in the virion interior interacts with the nucleocapsid. The nucleocapsid consists of the positive strand genomic RNA, mRNA, and the N protein region that interacts with the C-terminus of the M protein.

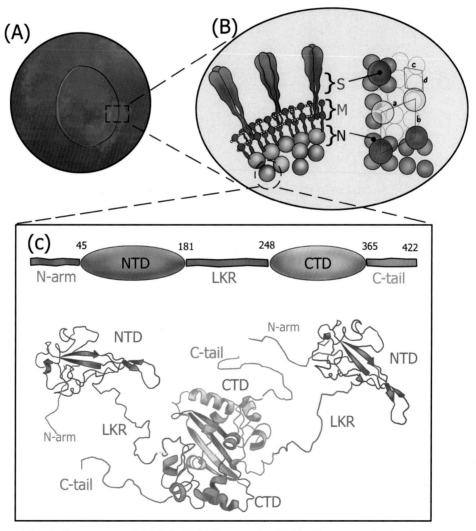

Fig. 1. Structure of SARS-CoV N-protein (C. K. Chang et al. 2006).

Fig. 1(A). 2D electron cryo-microscopy reconstructed image of SARS-CoV particle.

(B). Interpretation of the virion structure. Edge view of the conserved structural proteins is shown on the left panel and the axial view is shown on the right panel. Trimeric spikes (S) are shaded in red membrane proteins (M) are in solid blue, and nucleoproteins (N) are shaded in violet.

(C). The modular structural organization of SARS-CoV N protein.

The ribbon representations of the structures of N-terminal domain of N protein (amino acid. 45–181) NTD (green).

C-terminal domain of N protein (a.a. 248–365) CTD (blue and gold).

Linker region of SARS-CoV N protein (a.a. 182–247 (LKR) are drawn randomly to reflect the dynamic nature of the N protein.

The ribbon structures were generated using PyMOL (The PyMOL Molecular Graphics System, Version 1.5.0.4 Schrödinger, LLC).

The M-N interaction should therefore constrain some N molecules in close apposition to the envelope. To characterize the M-N interaction, density was plotted as a function of radial distance relative to the viral membrane.

Coronavirus assembly is localized at membranes of the endoplasmic reticulum-Golgi intermediate compartment and is mediated by species-specific interactions of the M protein with S, N, and envelope (E) proteins.

The stringency of structural protein organization at the site of budding is such that some transmembrane host proteins resident at the site of assembly are excluded from the virion, presumably due to tight M-M interactions (C. K. Chang et al. 2006).

Function of the SARS-CoV nucleocapsid (N) protein: The primary role of CoV N protein is to package the genomic viral genome into long, flexible, helical ribonucleoprotein (RNP) complexes called nucleocapsids or capsids.

1. **N is involved in the replication and budding of SARS-CoV at early time points of infection.**

The viral nucleocapsid protein, viral RNA, and the non-structural protein 3 (nsp3) are associated with characteristic membrane tubules and double-membrane vesicles that most probably originated from endoplasmic reticulum cisternae.

Experiments were carried out with Vero cells by infecting them with either mock or SARS-CoV for 3h or 5h. Cells were analyzed by immunofluorescence using antibodies against SARS-CoV N, SARS-CoV nsp3, or SARS –CoV S protein.

In summary, the immunofluorescence studies have shown that as early as 3 hours post-infection (h p.i.), cytoplasmic accumulations of SARS-CoV N are formed in infected cells which colocalize with SARS-CoV nsp3 and viral genomic RNA.

This suggested that viral nucleocapsid protein is the assembly and budding sites of the replication and budding of SARS-CoV.

2. **N protein of SARS-CoV in association with human Elongation Factor 1-alfa (EF1α) inhibits cytokinesis**: Experiments with yeast showed that the C terminus (amino acids 251 to 422) of the N protein interact with human elongation factor 1-alpha (EF1α), an essential component of the translational machinery with an important role in cytokinesis, promoting the bundling of filamentous actin (F-actin). In vitro and in vivo interaction was then confirmed by immuno-coprecipitation, far-Western blotting, and surface plasmon resonance. It was demonstrated that the N protein of SARS-CoV induces aggregation of EF1α, inhibiting protein translation and cytokinesis.

Interaction of N protein with EF1α was revealed by a yeast two-hybrid system. Three transformants containing pGBKT7-N and pACT2-EF1α(291-463) (left panel) together with both positive (upper right) and negative (lower right) controls were inoculated on SD-Leu⁻ Trp⁻ His⁻ Ade⁻-X-α-Gal plates. Transformants containing pGADT7-T and pGBKT7-p53 were used as a positive control, and transformants containing pGADT7-T and a pGBKT7-Lam were employed as a negative control.

EF1α in its GTP-bound form escorts aminoacyl-tRNA to ribosomes and plays an important role in protein synthesis. N protein of SARS-CoV associates with EF1α directly and induces EF1α aggregation. Because protein translation and cytokinesis were blocked by the expression of N protein, cell proliferation was inhibited.

During the development of a DNA vaccine against SARS-CoV, it was found that cytokinesis was blocked by the expression of the N protein of SARS-CoV in several cell lines. In addition, pathogenesis at the site of the intramuscular injection of mice following administration of an N protein expression plasmid was noted.

3. **N protein of SARS-CoV functions as interferon antagonist:** It has been determined that the high pathogenicity of SARS-CoV is because it antagonizes the function of interferon, a key component of the innate immune response.

N protein of SARs-CoV was expressed in Human Lung Cells (A549). The cell culture was obtained from American Type Culture Collection (ATCC), Manassas, VA, USA.

The A549 cells were transfected with plasmids containing expressing Ha-tagged SARS-CoV proteins. Hemagglutinin (HA) is a surface glycoprotein require for the infectivity.

At 24 h posttransfection, cells were infected with NDV-GFP plasmid (Newcastle Disease Virus-Green Fluorescence Protein).

Human Lung Cells (A549) were transfected with control or HA-tagged SARS-CoV plasmids.

(A). 24 h posttransfection, cells were infected with NDV-GFP, which grows in the presence of interferon antagonists. Images were obtained at 24 h postinfection using a 10× objective and are representative of three experiments.

(B). A549 cells were transfected with plasmids expressing HA-tagged SARS-CoV proteins for 24 h, fixed, and analyzed for expression of the SARS-CoV proteins using an antibody to the HA tag.

As shown in fig.8, all three proteins; SARS-CoV open reading frame (ORF) 3b, ORF 6, and N proteins antagonize interferon, a key component of the innate immune response.

SARS-CoV-2 infection generates innate immune responses: In the absence of preexisting specific (adaptive) immunity, the specific antigens of SARS-CoV-2 are not recognized. The innate immunity is the more rapid nonspecific responses to infection, such as surface defenses, cytokine production, complement activation and phagocytic responses.

These innate immune mechanisms and their interactions in defense against infection provide the host with the time needed to mobilize the more slowly developing mechanisms of adaptive immunity, which might protect against subsequent challenges.

The coronavirus SARS-CoV-2 uses its spike surface proteins to infect human cells. Spike proteins are heavily modified with several *N*-glycans, which are predicted to modulate their function. Interfering with either the synthesis or attachment of spike *N*-glycans significantly reduces the spread of SARS-CoV-2 infection *in vitro*, including that of several variants.

New SARS-CoV-2 variants, with various degrees of resistance against current vaccines, are likely to continue appearing.

CHAPTER 11

ECONOMIC IMPACT OF SARS-COV-2

The coronavirus 2019 disease (COVID-19) pandemic has created public health crisis and economic crisis worldwide. The economic crisis is unprecedented in its scale: the pandemic has created a demand shock, a supply shock, and a financial shock all at once.

Global stock markets erased about US$6 trillion in wealth in one week from 24th to 28th of February. The S&P 500 index lost over $5 trillion in value in the same week in the US while the S&P 500's largest 10 companies experienced a combined loss of over $1.4 trillion. (https://www.brookings.edu/research/ten-facts-about-covid-19-and-the-u-s-economy/, 2021).

COVID-19 has caused havoc in the whole world and has changed the world economy (fig.1).

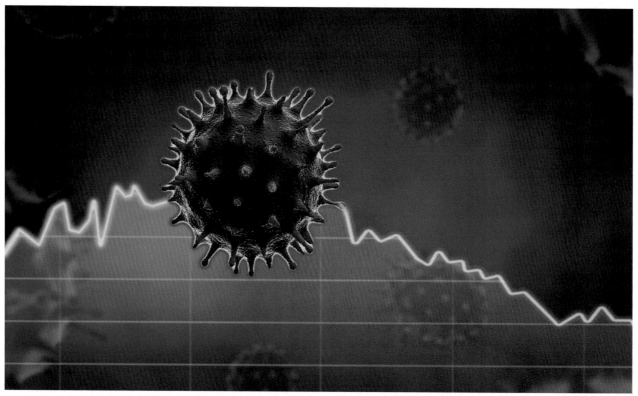

Fig.1. Coronavirus: How the pandemic has changed the world economy (L. Jones et al. 2021).

"The coronavirus pandemic has reached almost every country in the world. Its spread has left national economies and businesses counting the costs, as governments struggle with new lockdown measures to tackle the spread of the virus. The Financial Times Stock Exchange (FTSE), Dow Jones Industrial Average and the Nikkei all saw huge falls as the number of Covid-19 cases grew in the first months of the crisis" (Source).

"The World Health Organization (WHO) first declared COVID-19 a global health emergency in January 2020; on March 11 it announced the viral outbreak was officially a pandemic, the highest level of health emergency" (Source).

Since then, the emergency evolved into a global public health and economic crisis that affected the $90 trillion global economy beyond anything experienced in nearly a century. (www.washingtonpost.com, 2020).

1. The economic impact is bi-directional for COVID-19. The economic impact of COVID-19 has both supply and demand effects. With regard to consumption, we have been facing changing consumer attitudes and marketing channels. At the beginning of the COVID-19 process, rising consumer demand has been encountered attached to stockpiling. But both the demand dynamics and consumption and purchasing attitudes have changed. Web-based online shopping tools have long been used all over the world.

"While employment is rising and strains on household budgets have eased in recent months, the employment rate remains below pre-pandemic levels, and millions still report that their households did not get enough to eat or are not caught up on rent payments. Families meet everyday challenges such as paying rent, putting food on the table, affording child care and preschool, securing health coverage, and paying for college" (Source).

"We are able to track the extent of the nation's progress against hardship. Thanks to nearly real-time data from the Census Bureau's Household Pulse Survey and other sources" (Center on Budget and Policy Priorities, https://www.cbpp.org, updated on Nov. 10, 2021).

2. The shutdown/lockdown of financial markets and businesses: The stock market has often been a barometer for the path of the pandemic, tumbling after concerning milestones, and rising on advancements of vaccinations and new treatments. But the two haven't always moved in lock step, and Wall Street's performance has at times disregarded the human toll of the pandemic as it instead zeroed in on other factors that could drive corporate profits, like low interest rates and government spending.

The economic effects of COVID-19 around the world

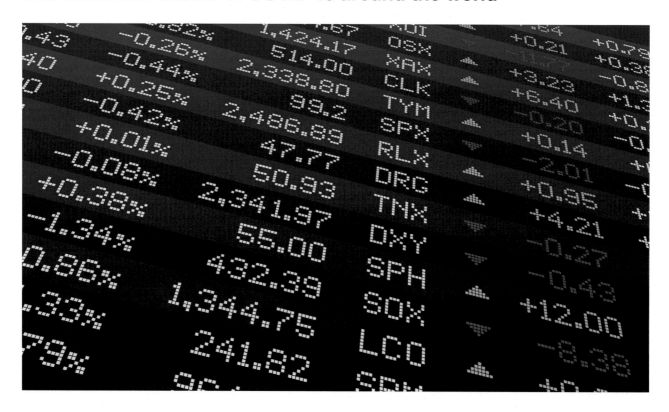

Fig. 2. New York Stock Exchange (www.weforum.org/12-14-21, image by Andrew Kelly, *Reuters*).

Economic effect of COVID-19 on New York Stock Exchange: "It's the latest round of market upheaval since the outbreak of Covid-19 roughly two years ago, with the virus repeatedly tilting Wall Street's assumptions about whether people would shop, travel or even turn up for work. Each new phase of the pandemic has brought new requirements for testing, border closings or warnings against public gatherings.

"The market's recoveries after pandemic-induced dips were underpinned by the Federal Reserve's measures to cut borrowing costs and keep capital pumping through the financial system. Progress on vaccines and other treatments helped mute market falls" (https://www.nytimes.com, December 7, 2021).

"The COVID-19 pandemic has spread with alarming speed infecting millions and bringing economic activity to a near-standstill as countries imposed tight restrictions on movement to halt the spread of virus" (www.worldbank. org, June 8, 2020).

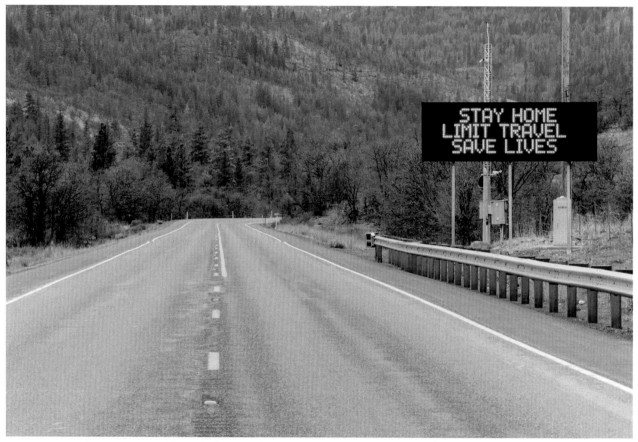

Fig. 3. An empty highway in Dubai during the coronavirus pandemic. Above the highway, a sign reads, "Stay Safe, Stay Home" (**Mo Azizi, Shutterstock).**

As the health and human toll grows, the economic damage is already evident and represents the largest economic shock the world has experienced in decades.

Global coordination and cooperation measures are needed to slow the spread of the pandemic, and of the economic actions needed to alleviate the economic damage.

Due to lockdown enforcement and voluntary social distancing, the service sector, restaurants, travel, tourism, catering, and leisure, got affected critically.

"Pandemic has hit the Restaurant Industry by changing the social norms. "Normally, change happens in an economic shock. This one just looks different. It came in the form of a pandemic instead of a housing crisis" (www.qsrmagazine.com, March 2021).

"Online-ordering platforms have watched demand for their services increase 10-fold since the start of the pandemic. As of mid-January, 89.6 percent of U.S. restaurants offered takeout, and 81.9 percent had delivery as an option, a third of which used three or more delivery apps. Fast-service restaurants were more likely to offer both takeout and delivery compared to their table-service counterparts" (www.qsrmagazine.com, March 2021).

"The International Air Transportation Association (IATA) expected passenger revenue loss for 2020 was $ 113 billion and this counts more than 20% of the overall projected revenue" (P. Ozili, T. Arun, 2020).

The airports are nearly empty as no passengers are traveling due to COVID-19 pandemic.

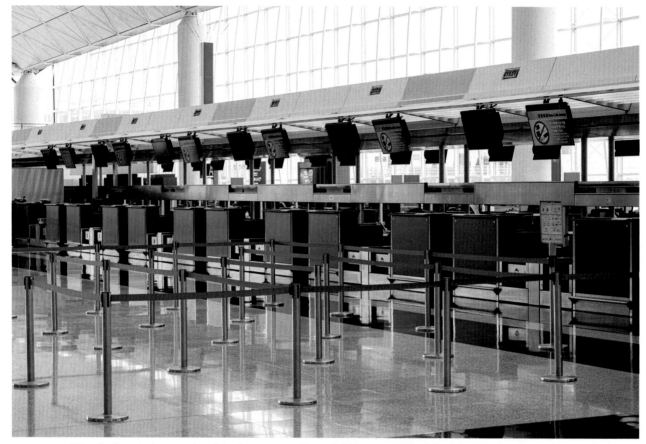

Fig. 4. A nearly empty view is seen at Ronald Reagan Washington National Airport, Arlington, Virginia (Alex Edelman, *AFP,* Getty Images, March 29, 2020).

The haunting photos of empty airports and planes at the height of the COVID-19 pandemic show the airline industry at its lowest point in decades (www.businessinsider.com, April 13, 2020)

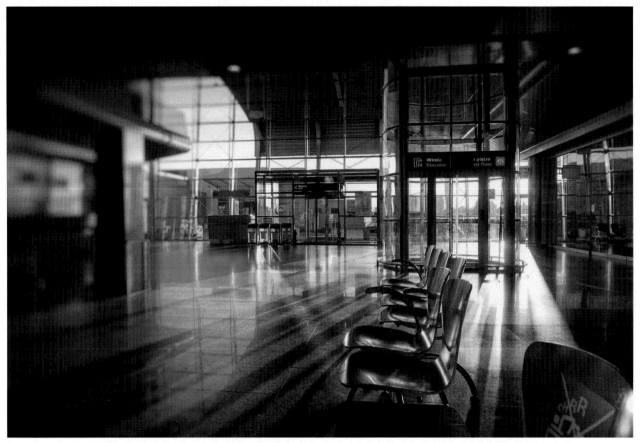

Fig. 5. Another example of a nearly empty view inside Chicago's O'Hare International Airport (Ryan Ewing, www.businessinsider.com, **April 13, 2020).**

The newly passed CARES Act requires airlines to maintain certain levels of pre-March 2020 air service even as passenger demand dwindles.

Despite the raging pandemic and stay at home orders, air travel remains the quickest form of transportation and is used by medical professionals and other essential workers to get where they're needed.

With non-essential travel limited, airports have become deserted and aircraft are flying with only handfuls of passengers if any.

Nowhere has the effect of COVID-19 been more pronounced in the US than the country's transportation system, especially its largest airports and the aircraft still flying.

Once vibrant, bustling centers for the facilitation of travel have been reduced to ghost towns operated by skeleton crews serving the few remaining flights that have yet to be cut by airlines.

Provisions of the Coronavirus Aid, Relief, and Economic Security Act, or the CARES Act, require of the airlines that apply for federal aid maintain minimal air service.

The law requires that airlines "maintain scheduled air transportation service as the Secretary of Transportation deems necessary to ensure services to any point served by that carrier before March 1, 2020."

Normally the third busiest airport in the US, Chicago's O'Hare International Airport is now a ghost town as the virus has decimated demand.

American Airlines has largely shifted to cargo-only flights from its New York gateway.

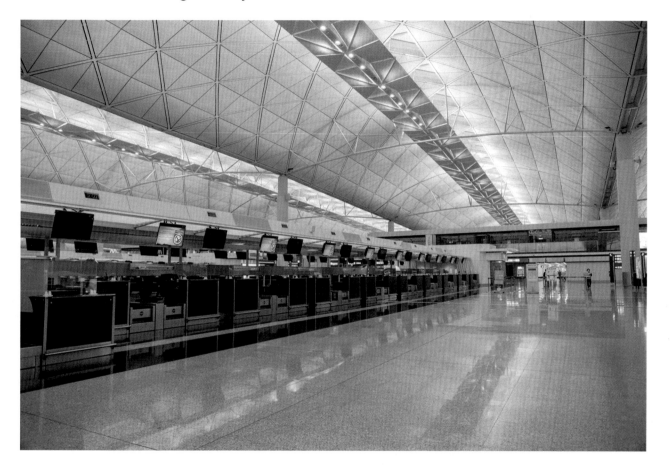

Fig. 6. Terminal 8 at New York's JFK Airport (James Charalambous,
www.businessinsider.com**, April 13, 2020).**

New York has been among the hardest-hit cities in the country, with around 6,000 deaths due to COVID-19 and nearly 200,000 reported cases statewide.

Even the country's busiest airport, Hartsfield-Jackson Atlanta International, is eerily quiet. Its largest carrier, Delta Air Lines, has shifted to cargo-only flights.

Ticket counters remain similarly empty and largely unstaffed as airlines offer voluntary layoffs for employees in an effort to preserve cash flow.

Empty flights are virtually guaranteed but airlines are required to keep flying some services under the CARES Act in order to receive federal funds.

Only 10 passengers took the near-3-hour journey from New York to Miami on this Boeing 777-200 capable of seating around 275.

Social distancing on these flights is more easily achieved with no shortage of empty seats and rows.

On this flight from Washington to New Orleans, only one passenger showed up to fly on this 70-seat regional jet (www. businessinsider.com, April 13, 2020).

The lockdown enforcement and declining demand are apparently leading to downsizing in all these industries.

The increasing number of lockdown days, monetary policy decisions, and international travel restrictions severely affected the level of economic activities and the closing, opening, lowest and highest stock price of major stock market indices.

In contrast, the imposed restriction on internal movement and higher fiscal policy spending had a positive impact on the level of economic activities.

Netherlands lockdown enforcements include closing bars, restaurants, and most stores from 5:00 p.m.–5:00 a.m. (*Reuters*, Dec 17).

Canada recorded a much smaller budget deficit in the first seven months of the 2021/22 fiscal year compared to the same period a year ago, as the costs of the COVID-19 crisis continued to recede, the finance ministry said on Friday (*Reuters*).

The April to October shortfall was C$72.25 billion ($56.29 billion) compared with a C$216.62 billion deficit over the same seven months in 2020/21, the data showed (*Reuters*).

3. Social distancing policies on economic activities and stock market indices: "A systematic search was carried out in eleven databases on social distancing. Papers were included in the review if they reported on qualitative studies of factors influencing the implementation of social distancing measures in potentially epidemic infectious diseases. An adapted meta-ethnographical approach was used for synthesis. Review findings were assessed for strength and reliability using GRADE-CERQual. The review identifies two broad categories of barriers to social distancing measures: individual- or community-level psychosocial phenomena, and shortcomings in governmental action or communication. Based on this, 25 themes are identified that can be addressed to improve the implementation of social distancing. They concluded that there are a range of barriers, on different levels, to the implementation of social distancing measures. There is a need for authorities to involve their communities and provide continuous support in adhering to social distancing, and developing measures that are necessary for the pandemic response. Policies should be designed with these factors in mind to ensure an effective, ethical and equitable pandemic response. The current situation further calls for high-quality research to better describe mechanisms by which acceptability and implementation of social distancing measures can be improved" (Source).

4. Shift in demand for production: There is less demand for services, such as retailing, aviation, leisure, and more demand for government support.

5. Spending and saving attitudes of consumers: "The bank transactions were evaluated to estimate spending and saving attitudes in the USA and results showed that consumer spending for necessities rose by 56% due stockpiling from the end of February to the mid of March" (Source).

6. Cyclical impact of rising unemployment: "The cyclical impact of rising unemployment seems to reduce all interior and international trade opportunities due to falling income and negatively shifting demand for most products.

"Some projections made by international organisations are overwhelming. International Labour Organisation (ILO) estimated 10.5% job deterioration for the second quarter of 2020 due to COVID-19, meaning loss of 309 million full-time jobs. The previous quarterly estimate was 195 million and the estimated unemployment rose by almost 60% by the mid of April 2020" (Source).

7. Uncertainty in investments and international trade: "The exponential rate the virus was spreading, and the heightened uncertainty, about how bad the situation could get led to safety in consumption and investment among consumers, investors and international trade partners.

"The Dow Jones Industrial Average Index (DJIA), along with other market indices, lost one-third of its value between February 14, 2022, and March 23, 2020. The Index rose steadily between March and November and rose nearly three percentage points on Monday, November 9, 2020, reportedly on news that a COVID-19 vaccine had been developed.

"The COVID-19 crisis also led to dramatic swings in household spending. Retail sales, which primarily tracks sales of consumer goods, declined 8.7 percent from February to March 2020, the largest month-to-month decrease since the Census Bureau started tracking the data" (US Census Bureau, 2020a).

Global International Trade is a part of global interconnectedness that comprises 4 distinct types of transactions: supply chains, capital, information, and people.

The pandemic affected cross-border movements of trade and people the most in response to travel restrictions, according to the December 2020 reports by DHL and the New York University, Stern Scholl of Business.

8._Efforts to ease the COVID-19 crisis: The International Recovery Platform (IRP) issued the COVID-19 Recovery Policy brief that states 8 principles as follows:

1. Recovery must begin during the ongoing response.

2_Inclusive, people-centered recovery to leave no one behind

3. Transparent evidence-based decision-making

4. Build back better (BBB) and greener

5. Preserve development gains

6. Greater regional and global solidarity

7. Institutionalize effective coping mechanisms

8. Effective risk communication

The federal fiscal policy of the USA response to the COVID-19 pandemic has taken two primary tasks;

1. aid to businesses.
2. aid to households and unemployed workers.

A series of laws, notably The Coronavirus Aid, Relief, and Economic Security Act (CARES) Act and the Families First Act were passed.

The CARES Act has provided relief to small businesses in terms of the Paycheck Protection Program (PPP). According to the Small Business Pulse Survey, 73.5 percent of small businesses surveyed requested financial assistance from the PPP; 25.6 percent requested economic injury disaster loans, and 13 percent requested small business administration loan forgiveness between March 13 and September 5.

The PPP was initially allocated $349 billion to offer loans to small businesses, with such loans being forgiven if businesses retained workers and maintained payroll. The program was significantly oversubscribed, and larger businesses disproportionately received funding. In particular, although loans for over $1 million only represented 4 percent of all loans processed in the first round of PPP, they represented 45 percent of all dollars disbursed. As a result, an additional $310 billion was allocated to the PPP, nearly half of which had been disbursed by early August; this second round resulted in a greater number of smaller loans to smaller businesses (L. Bauer et al. 2020).

The Family First Act provided an unprecedented level of federal resources to households, largely through one-time stimulus payments and expanded unemployment insurance (UI) payments. As a result of those payments, disposable personal income was nearly 10 percent higher in the second quarter of 2020 relative to the first quarter, even though employee compensation fell almost 7 percent This Bureau of Economic Analysis webpage consolidated information about the COVID-19 virus and federal stimulus programs (Bureau of Economic Analysis [BEA], US Department of Commerce, 2020).

.The Families First Act and CARES Act included stimulus payments for households based on income, expanded unemployment insurance (UI) eligibility, an increase of $600 in UI payments to recipients.

The Supplemental Nutrition Assistance Program (SNAP) is the largest Federal Nutrition Assistance Program that provides an electronic benefits transfer card to purchase eligible food from authorized retail food stores.

While employment is rising and strains on household budgets have eased in recent months, the employment rate remains below pre-pandemic levels, and millions still report that their households did not get enough to eat or are not caught up on rent payments. We are able to track the extent of the nation's progress against hardship. Thanks to nearly real-time data from the Census Bureau's Household Pulse Survey and other sources (Center on Budget and Policy Priorities (https://www.cbpp.org, updated on November 10, 2021).

Build Back Better, the Federal Aid Project, if passed, would help Americans in 5 key areas:

1. This bill includes funding for new Housing Choice vouchers for roughly 300,000 households with the lowest incomes.
2. This bill will extend through 2022 the American Rescue Plan's expansion of the earned income tax credit.

3. This bill will increase access to affordable child care and enable workers to take paid time off from work to care for a new child or an ill loved one or to attend to their own health issues.

   The bill also includes substantial investments to make college more affordable and accessible and to expand workforce development opportunities that help people develop skills for in-demand jobs, investments that can reduce student debt, improve job prospects, and boost the nation's productivity.

4. The Build Back Better would raise revenues to finance its investments and would make our tax system fairer. The bill would shrink tax breaks for the wealthy households and profitable corporations and give Internal Revenue Services (IRS) resources so that it can do more to ensure that individuals and corporations pay what they legally owe. These revenue provisions, coupled with the bill's provisions that would reduce the cost of prescription drugs, are important policy advances on their own and would provide needed resources to finance the bill's investments.

   The fiscal impact of Build Back Better is roughly zero over the next decade and around $2 trillion in deficit reduction in the subsequent decade.

5. The Build Back Better would reduce racial disparities and expand protections for immigrants. The investments in Build Back Better would provide health coverage and access, housing, and education stemming from generations of racism and other forms of discrimination.

Build Back Better would make transformational investments in children, families, workers, climate, and health coverage (https://www.bbc.com/news/business-51706225).

The IMF has secured $1 trillion in lending capacity, serving members and responding fast to an unprecedented number of emergency financing requests from over 90 countries so far (www.imf.org, 2021).

In the early stages of the global economic recession, economic forecasts were compounded further by a historic drop in the price of crude oil. Since then, oil prices recovered from the low of nearly $20 per barrel in April 2020 to a range of $40–$45 per barrel by the end of 2020, in part reflecting the decline in global economic activity. By early June 2021, the international price had crossed the $70 per barrel mark, where it remained through early October when it rose above $80 dollars per barrel. Through the first half of 2021, economic forecasts turned more positive based on an expected return to pre-pandemic rates of growth" (www.washingtonpost.com, March 4, 2020).

The WHO indicated that the USA was experiencing the third wave of infections as a result of Delta and Omicron variants.

"China emerged in June 2020 as the first major country to announce a return to economic growth since the COVID-19 pandemic. China is still grappling with the economic effects of the COVID-19 pandemic, however, including sluggish domestic consumption, slow recovery in its top export markets, and reliance on government spending and exports to boost initial growth" (*In Focus* [2021], https://crsreports.congress.gov).

Despite the pandemic recession, personal bankruptcies actually declined dramatically throughout the past two years. Close observers say that's because government programs like increased unemployment insurance and the eviction moratorium kept lots of people afloat, at least enough to avoid bankruptcy.

CHAPTER 12

MENTAL-HEALTH EFFECT OF SARS-COV-2

It is no surprise that mental health problems went up during the COVID-19 pandemic. The hospitalization surge is unprecedented in this pandemic. Physical activity is critical to good health; if you have a chronic health condition like liver, kidney, or heart disease, or diabetes, all of which have shown to lead to worse outcomes in people battling the virus.

Anxiety and depression are increasing as the pandemic goes on. Numerous studies have documented mental health challenges during the COVID-19 pandemic.

Mental health affects how we think (cognitive), feel (psychological), and act (behavioral).

Mental health also helps determine how we handle stress, relate to others, and make choices. Each of these components interacts with and influences the others, and they are all imperative to overall well-being.

Mental health is not something you have, it is something you practice.

Mental health includes three major components (www.mentalhealth.gov, USA, 2021).

3 Components of Mental Health

> cognitive
> psychological
> behavioral

Cognitive: Cognitive "refers to 'the mental action or process of acquiring knowledge and understanding through thought, experience, and the senses'. It encompasses many aspects of intellectual functions and processes such as: perception, attention, the formation of knowledge, memory and working memory, judgment and evaluation, reasoning and 'computation', problem solving and decision making, comprehension and production of language. Cognitive processes use existing knowledge and discover new knowledge" (https://en.wikipedia.org, accessed on November 11, 2021).

Psychological: "Psychological are emotional states brought on by neurophysiological changes, variously associated with thoughts, feelings, behavioural responses, and a degree of pleasure or displeasure" (Source).

"Psychological or emotional health is an important part of overall health. People who are emotionally healthy are in control of their thoughts, feelings, and behaviours. It means you're aware of your emotions. You can deal with them, whether they're positive or negative. Emotionally healthy people still feel stress, anger, and sadness" (Source).

Behavioral: "Behavioral is the range of actions and mannerisms made by individuals, organisms, systems or artificial entities in conjunction with themselves or their environment, which includes the other systems or organisms around as well as the physical environment" (https://en.wikipedia. org, accessed on November 11, 2021).

Mental health and clinical medicine as interdisciplinary approach to the COVID-19 pandemic: The new research could develop data that combines mental health and medicine in combating the pandemic situations such as the ongoing COVID-19 pandemic.

"The COVID-19 pandemic is having alarming implications for individual and collective health and emotional and social functioning. Health care providers have an additional role in monitoring psychological needs and delivering psychological support to their patients. The Covid-19 pandemic has awakened many physicians to the value of viewing wellness and disease through the lens of public health as well as that of clinical medicine. To help foster such a reframing, a Perspective series, entitled "Fundamentals of Public Health" has been launched in the *New England Journal of Medicine*" (*N Eng J Med*)" (Source).

Effect of physical distancing on mental health: To reduce the spread of the virus, physical distancing was an important step taken to protect self and others. Physical distancing is a prevention method to slow the person-to-person transmission of COVID-19.

In public health, social distancing, also called physical distancing, is a set of non-pharmaceutical interventions or measures intended to prevent the spread of a contagious disease by maintaining a physical distance between people and reducing the number of times people come into close contact with each other. It usually involves keeping a certain distance from others and avoiding gathering together in large groups.

Physical distancing had negative impacts on the mental health of individuals and communities. It caused fear and anxiety and had financial ramifications. Physical distancing involved a range of restrictions that affected the daily lives of the people. School closings were perceived as having the strongest effect on daily lives and psychological outcomes (CDC.gov, USA, 2021).

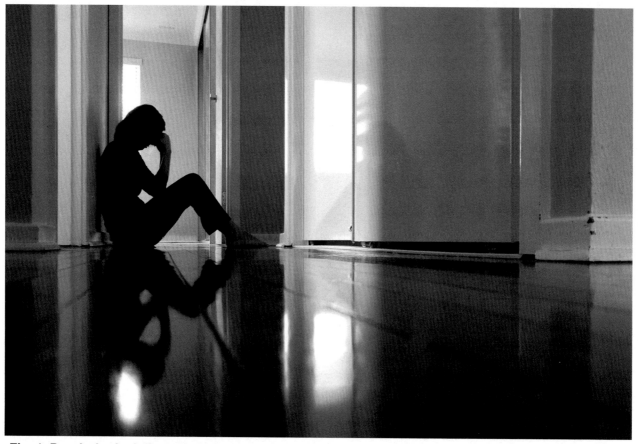

Fig. 1. Psychological distress during the pandemic, especially anxiety (www.shutterlock.com, 2021).

Effect of quarantine on mental health: Quarantine is the separation and restriction of movement of people who have potentially been exposed to a contagious disease to ascertain if they become unwell, so reducing the risk of them infecting others This definition differs from isolation, which is the separation of people who have been diagnosed with a contagious disease from people who are not sick; however, the two terms are often used interchangeably, especially in communication with the public.

The word quarantine was first used in Venice, Italy in 1127 with regard to leprosy and was widely used in response to the Black Death, although it was not until 300 years later that the UK properly began to impose quarantine in response to the plague. This outbreak has seen entire cities in China effectively placed under mass quarantine, while many thousands of foreign nationals returning home from China have been asked to self-isolate at home or in state-run facilities. Citywide quarantines were also imposed in areas of China and Canada during the 2003 outbreak of severe acute respiratory syndrome (SARS), whereas entire villages in many West African countries were quarantined during the 2014 Ebola outbreak. Quarantine is often an unpleasant experience for those who undergo it. Separation from loved ones, the loss of freedom, uncertainty over disease status, and boredom can, on occasion, create dramatic effects. Suicide has been reported in several cases. Professional mental health support needs to be offered to avoid such happenings.

Successful use of quarantine as a public health measure requires us to reduce, as far as possible, the negative effects associated with it.

Quarantine could be a double-edged sword; while it is effective in the containment of COVID-19, it has profound negative effects on individual lives, travel, and well-being.

A systematic review was conducted in order to identify (i) the social consequences of mass quarantine during infectious disease outbreaks and (ii) recommend strategies to mitigate the negative social implications of COVID-19 movement restrictions. Eleven articles from various geographical and disease contexts highlighted the psychological implications of mass quarantine as emotional distress and symptoms of mental illness. Among people in or after quarantine, some experienced emotional distress, including: annoyance, anxiety, boredom, disappointment and life dissatisfaction, fear of infection, loneliness and mistrust.

During the COVID-19 lockdown, there was strong evidence that those who stopped working had poorer mental health conditions than those still employed [a decrease of 2.60 points in Mental Composite Scale; 95% confidence interval (CI) = −0.05 to −5.16]. While one study revealed that people under physical distancing and movement restrictions suffered insomnia and depression.

Stress in the current pandemic: Stress is a crucial component of mental health and relates to the prevalence of anxiety and depression in the general population during the COVID-19 pandemic. A systematic review and meta-analysis focused on stress and anxiety prevalence among the general population during the COVID-19 pandemic was conducted. Data were searched in the Science Direct, Embase, Scopus, PubMed, Web of Science and Google Scholar databases, without a lower time limit and until May 2020. In order to perform a meta-analysis of the collected studies, the random effects model was used, and the heterogeneity of studies was investigated using the I^2 index. Data analysis was conducted using the Comprehensive Meta-Analysis (CMA) software. The results obtained revealed the prevalence of stress in 5 studies with a total sample size of 9074 as 29.6% (95% confidence limit: 24.3–35.4), the prevalence of anxiety in 17 studies with a sample size of 63,439 as 31.9% (95% confidence interval:

27.5–36.7), and the prevalence of depression in 14 studies with a sample size of 44,531 people as 33.7% (95% confidence interval: 27.5–40.6).

It was concluded that COVID-19 not only causes physical health concerns but also results in a number of psychological disorders. The spread of the new coronavirus can impact the mental health of people in different communities. Thus, it is essential to preserve the mental health of individuals and to develop psychological interventions that can improve the mental health of vulnerable groups during the COVID-19 pandemic.

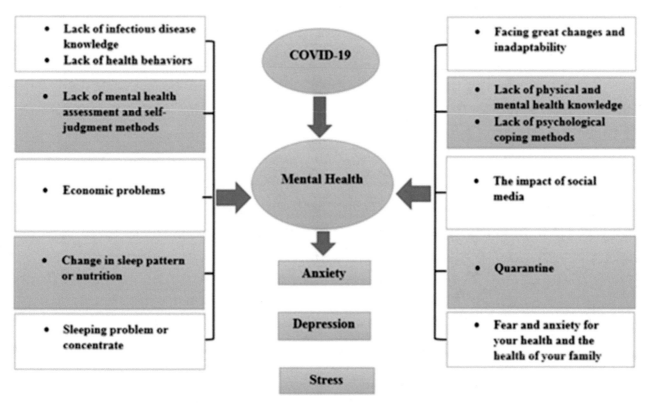

Fig. 2. Effect of COVID-19 on mental health resulting in anxiety, depression, and stress (N. Salari et al. 2020).

Although COVID-19 is a new strain of coronaviruses, it is known that coronaviruses cause diseases ranging from cold to more severe illnesses such as SARS and MERS. Symptoms of the Coronavirus infection include fever, chills, cough, sore throat, myalgia, nausea and vomiting, and diarrhea. Men with a history of underlying diseases are more likely to be infected with the virus and would experience worse outcomes. Generalized anxiety disorder, depressive symptoms, and sleep quality during the COVID-19 epidemic have been reported.

The COVID-19 pandemic has affected mental health in all contexts and has highlighted the weaknesses of mental health systems globally. COVID-19 has shown the mental health impacts of pandemics not only on individuals with existing mental health needs but also across populations due to the policies aimed to stem its spread, which disproportionately affects vulnerable and already disadvantaged groups.

The rapid spread of the infection and the severity of COVID-19 caused a partial collapse of the sanitary systems in many countries of the world. The fatigue, fear of getting sick, fear for one's family, precarious organization, and preventive isolation might also contribute to cause mental illness. The participating doctors felt nervous after listening to the news on mass media that some doctors were positive for COVID-19, whereas 52.6% of the participating nurses report negative emotion, worrying about family, fear of infection, and stress about a heavy workload.

The COVID-19 pandemic has had a strong impact on healthcare workers (HCWs), affecting their physical and mental health. In Italy, HCWs have been among the first exposed to unprecedented pressure, dealing with large numbers of infections during the first pandemic wave. However, the severe psychological consequences on HCWs find little evidence in the literature, especially in terms of comparison to the status quo before pandemic.

Psychological effects of the pandemic on people with pre-existing medical conditions:

The undesirable COVID-19 health outcomes have consistently increased in certain patient subgroups. The pre-existing health conditions and the strength of associations differ between the geographical regions. In order to find the associations between multiple pre-existing health conditions and clearly defined COVID-19 outcomes, a study was conducted using an umbrella review approach.

"The umbrella review is a systematic collection and assessment of evidence reported in systematic literature reviews. The methods of umbrella review allow for the analysis of a large body of evidence on the strength of associations and confidence in the estimates. The umbrella reviews have been more frequently used to synthesize available evidence and inform clinical practice. The umbrella review methodology was applied for this study because it allowed us to systematically and efficiently compile the published evidence on associations between a broad spectrum of pre-existing conditions and several COVID-19 outcomes across geographical regions into a single informative review.

The study protocol was registered in the International Prospective Register of Systematic Reviews (PROSPERO; registration no. CRD42020215846)" (Source).

In the COVID-19 pandemic, individuals with chronic pre-existing health conditions are potentially at higher risk for disease progression to severe stages requiring hospitalisation and intensive care and leading to death. However, the occurrence of severe cases in older age groups suggests that the effect of age on poor COVID-19 outcomes is more pronounced.

The results of this review show that heart failure, obesity, diabetes, liver cirrhosis, chronic kidney disease, active and haematological cancer, and history of organ transplantation are associated with an increased risk of poor COVID-19-related outcomes such as hospitalisation, need for intensive care and death. The causal effects of the pre-existing conditions were not identified, but rather to summarise the evidence on the diseases associated with the worsening of COVID-19. However, regional heterogeneity observed for multiple associations suggests an influence of other factors outside the scope of this review. For example, the association between HIV and COVID-19-related mortality was stronger in the African region than in the European region and North America. Prevalent progressed stages of HIV, poor nutritional status and limited access to antiviral treatment are likely to strengthen the association between HIV and COVID-19-related morality in the African region. Further epidemiological studies conducted in different areas are needed to untangle the effects of potential confounding factors and to estimate the causal effects of pre-existing health conditions. (Source)

Burnout and posttraumatic stress disorder in the COVID-19 pandemic: "(COVID-19) pandemic has presented myriad challenges to the health care system. Health care providers are facing unprecedented acute workplace stress compounded by a high baseline rate of physician burnout. In health care, this circumstance is so profound that the COVID-19 pandemic has required an adoption of the language of war. There is talk of physician redeployment to the frontline and sophisticated statistics track daily causalities while military style temporary hospitals are constructed. CNN has compared the epidemic's impact on our civilization to that of World War II.

Symptoms related to PTSD fall into three categories that include reliving the event, a sense of emotional numbness or depersonalization, and symptoms of increased arousal (difficulty sleeping, feeling irritated or easily angered). Additionally, because there are significant overlaps in drivers of both PTSD and burnout, as well as consequences and comorbidities, the intersection of these entities may have a compounding effect" (Source).

Burnout is a psychological syndrome described as a self-reported state of care- or work-related physical and mental stress that induces emotional exhaustion, depersonalization, and a sense of reduced personal accomplishment. Burnout is defined as "a syndrome of exhaustion, depersonalization, and reduced professional efficacy". Burnout is composed of two elements: "exhaustion", linked to excessive job demands; and "disengagement", linked to insufficient job resources.

Burnout was first applied to healthcare workers (HCWs) by Freudenberger in 1974. Due to substantial disagreement in the health literature on what exactly constitutes burnout and therefore on how to measure it, there is a great heterogeneity in the prevalence of this phenomenon.

In the current period of global public health crisis due to the COVID-19, healthcare workers are more exposed to physical and mental exhaustion. The very high number of cases and deaths, and the probable future "waves" raise awareness of these challenging working conditions and the need to address burnout by identifying possible solutions.

Traumatic events or adverse conditions during natural disasters, and pandemics may lead to burnout.

During the severe acute respiratory syndrome (SARS), H1N1, and Ebola outbreaks, studies showed that frontline HCWs were at higher risk of developing psychological sequelae, including chronic stress, anxiety, depression and post-traumatic stress disorder. Various factors are understood to have contributed to this phenomenon, such as excessive workload, concerns about occupational exposure, or infection of HCWs' families. In comparison to previous pandemics, the psychological impact of COVID-19 may be more significant and widespread, given the scale of the pandemic.

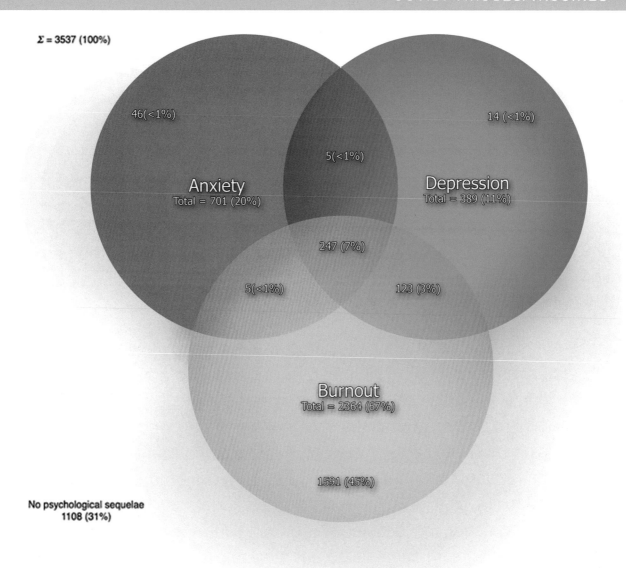

Σ = 3537 (100%)

46(<1%)

5(<1%)

14 (<1%)

Anxiety
Total = 701 (20%)

Depression
Total = 389 (11%)

247 (7%)

5(<1%)

123 (3%)

Burnout
Total = 2364 (67%)

1591 (45%)

No psychological sequelae
1108 (31%)

**Fig. 3. Venn diagram demonstrating the prevalence of anxiety,
depression, and burnout in the sampled population.**

Burnout, anxiety, and depression have a negative impact on staff and patient outcomes as well as lead to workforce attrition.

Effects of COVID-19 on healthcare workers (HCWs) and on healthcare systems:

A first direct effect of burnout is, of course, on HCWs' own care and safety. The rate of depressive disorder among HCWs is alarming when compared with that of the general population and is closely related to high levels of occupational stress. During the COVID-19 outbreak, a relatively high prevalence of anxiety (24.94%), depression (24.83%) and sleep disorders (44.03%) was reported in meta-analyses investigating the mental health of HCWs. Healthcare workers tend to hide their difficulties due to the perceived stigma associated with mental illness as well as to the fear of an impact on their careers.

These mental conditions are associated with further criticalities, including a 25% increased odds of alcohol abuse or dependence and a doubled risk of suicidal ideation. When considering the extreme act, it is well known that the rates are higher among physicians than in the general populations. An overall standardized mortality rate for suicide in physicians has been reported as 1.44, with a higher level in females as 1.99. They also found a higher risk for anesthesiologists, psychiatrists, general practitioners and general surgeons. Although, at present, no data sets regarding the impact of COVID-19 on physician mental health and suicide are available, the many news published in the newspapers of various countries about the suicide of doctors active in the pandemic leave no doubt that the situation is getting worse.

Burnout is a critical issue that generates inefficiency in healthcare organizations. The economic cost of physicians' reduced wellbeing can be mainly assessed in terms of the organizational cost of replacing them, decreased productivity and other "blind" issues. These costs have been estimated to be between $ 500,000 and $ 1,000,000 for replacing a single physician with the invaluable training and experience consequently lost. Moreover, they reported a 30% reduction in work effort for each 1-point increase in burnout (on a 7-point scale), and highlighted other costs arising from losing mentors for junior faculty and grants, or from managing medical errors and complaints of negligence.

Measures to mitigate burnout and harm arising from psychological distress following the Covid-19 pandemic: "Mental disorders have multiple determinants; prevention needs to be a multipronged effort. Implementation should be guided by available evidence. Measures have been suggested to prevent or reduce burnout" (who.int/mental_health, accessed on November 11, 2021).

Physical activity: Physical activity and exercise can be very effective in relieving stress. Just going out and getting some fresh air, like going for a walk to the shops can really help.

Balanced diet: Eating healthily provides adequate amounts of nutrition; essential vitamins and minerals and water to the brain that can improve the feelings of well-being. It could reduce the risks of malnutrition that could be devastating to an individual's health. I could reduce burnout and psychological stress during the COVID-19 pandemic.

Substance use: Substance use refers to smoking, vaping (Tobacco or marijuana), and heavy alcohol use. Substance use could increase the risk of more severe symptoms of mental distress and a higher risk of death if a person contracts COVID-19. Avoid substance use and get help from the health provider.

Relax: Relax by using meditation techniques and deep breathing exercises. It could reduce burnout and stress. Strike the balance between responsibility to others and responsibility to self, which can really reduce stress levels.

Be mindful: "Mindfulness is a mind-body approach to life that helps to relate differently to experiences. It involves paying attention to our thoughts and feelings in a way that increases our ability to manage difficult situations and make wise choices. Try to practice mindfulness regularly. Mindfulness meditation can be practiced anywhere at any time. Research has suggested that it can reduce the effects of stress, anxiety and related problems such as insomnia, poor concentration and low moods. The website, Be Mindful, features online courses in mindfulness to help in the COVID-19 situation" (Source).

Pandemic related changes in psychological stress: Numerous studies have documented mental health challenges during the COVID-19 pandemic. Few studies included pre-pandemic levels of mental health or were comprehensive in assessing factors likely associated with longer-term mental health impacts.

SARS-CoV-2 has been strongly associated with an increased risk of mental health. Cardiovascular and cerebrovascular diseases share the same set of risk factors, and are important prognostic factors for poor outcome in COVID-19 infections.

Risk of COVID complications was examined using psychological distress (anxiety and depression) as predictors by statistical analysis of a large amount of data obtained from several subsets of participants in the nationwide Cancer Prevention Study-3 (CPS-3) United States cohort (N=2,359; 1,534 women; 825 men) who completed surveys in 2018 and during the COVID-19 pandemic (July–September 2020). Table 1 shows the results of COVID complications.

Table 1: Predictors of Anxiety and Depression Stratified by Sex: Logistic Regression

	WomenOR (95% CI)	MenOR (95% CI)
Age (continuous)	1.00 90.99-1.010	0.99 (0.97-1.01)
Race		
Non-Hispanic White	1	1
Other	0.89 (0.71-1.11)	0.66 (0.41-1.05)
Predictor: Risk of COVID complications		
Low risk	1	1
Increased risk	1.75 (1.13-2.71)	2.47 (0.93-6.57)

Among women only, the odds of psychological distress were lower for those who were at increased risk for COVID-19 complications (OR=1.75; 95% CI: 1.13-2.71).

In men only, the odds of psychological distress (OR = 2.47; 95% CI: (0.93 – 6.57) at 95% CI) was lower than women.

OR stands for Odd Ratios, CI stands for Confidence Intervals.

All Multivariate ordinal logistic regression models were stratified by sex and the statistical analyses were performed with SAS 9.4 Software.

Ordinal variable: This is special semi-quantitative type of categorical variable where the values are conceptually ordered, such as degree of pain (e.g. none, mild, moderate, severe) or psychological distress.

Odds ratio (OR) for a specified response: For a binary explanatory variable, the OR is calculated as the odds of the specified response in those with the explanatory feature, divided by the odds of that response in those without the explanatory feature. If there is truly no association then the two odds should be approximately equal and the OR approximately 1, which is therefore the value for a 'null association'

Logistic regression: This is a method for analysis of the occurrence or not of a particular response value, in relation to potential explanatory variables. What is modelled for each combination of explanatory variables is the logarithm of the odds of that response value (which is termed a logistic transformation). Each association in the model is summarised/estimated in terms of an odds ratio (OR).

CHAPTER 13

TESTING FOR SARS-COV-2

COVID-19 infections are spreading and it is affecting different people in different ways.

Coronavirus disease (COVID-19) is an infectious disease caused by the SARS-CoV-2 virus.

Anyone who has symptoms of COVID-19 infection or is at high risk of exposure to SARS-CoV-2 should be tested for SARS-CoV-2.

There are diagnostic tests for SARS-CoV-2, such as nucleic acid amplification test (NAAT), and Antigen Tests.

Diagnostic tests have been authorized for use by trained personnel in several settings, including lab facilities. They can also be used in point-of-care settings, where the test is performed by trained personnel at or near the place where the specimen was collected. Point-of-care settings include physician offices, pharmacies, long-term care facilities, and school clinics.

Testing for COVID-19 detects the current infection with the virus and allows us to make a decision for the emergency response if the test is positive.

Negative test results at a single point in time warrants re-test using a gold standard option. It can take days from when you were actually exposed to the coronavirus to the point at which it is built up enough in your body for even the gold standard tests to detect. If you are symptomatic but test negative, it is still possible you have COVID, so should take extra precautions.

The Biden administration is providing 10 million COVID-19 tests/month to schools across the country (www.cnn.org, Jan 12, 2022).

According to the administration, 96% of schools in the country are currently open ("Statements and Releases," www.whitehouse.gov, January 14, 2022) compared with 46 percent of schools in January 2021.

It is estimated that about 5,000–10,000 US schools either shifted to virtual classes or closed temporarily. The administration announced test-to-stay strategy that aims to keep students in school. Test-to-stay (TTS) strategy means that school-associated people (Students, Staff, and other workers) can stay in the school, if tested negative (asymptomatic), and the school can be open.

Test-to-stay can be resource intensive because testing involves equipment and chemicals. It may not be a viable option for every school. The local public health agencies have to comply with all the applicable laws, regulations, and policies so that the learning goes on with minimum disruption.

In light of the updated data, CDC has added information on test-to-stay practices to K12 webpages. The K12 web pages have information on prevention (masks) and vaccination. It requires everyone age 2 and older to wear a mask inside schools and facilities, keep at least 3 feet distance between individuals, screening testing, ventilation, handwashing, and staying home when sick ("Guidance for COVID-19 prevention in K-12 schools," www. CDC.gov, updated on January 13, 2022).

Adolescents ages 16 years and older can get a booster shot at least six months after a primary series. Widespread vaccination for COVID-19 is a critical tool to best protect everyone from COVID-19 and COVID-19-related complications.

Test-to-stay combines contact tracing and serial testing.

Contact tracing: Close contacts that had a prior infection help to trace the transmission of COVID-19.

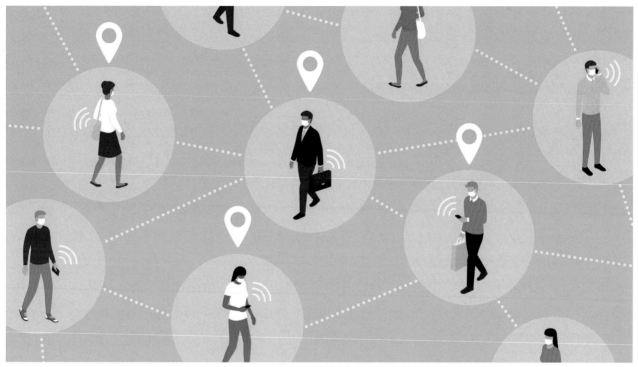

Fig.1. Contact tracing ("Toolkit for Responding to COVID-19 Cases," www.cdc.gov, updated on December 28, 2021)

Serial testing: Serial testing means testing the same person repeatedly. The testing is repeated at least twice during a seven-day period after the last close contact with a person with COVID-19. Testing frequency after close contact can vary (for example, from twice in a seven-day period to daily). More frequent testing can more quickly identify students who become infected with COVID-19.

Regular testing: Testing is offered regularly to all people even to those who don't have symptoms of COVID-19. Regular testing is done with written consent. Minors will not be tested without the consent of both the Minor and the Minor's guardian.

Regular testing, in addition to COVID-19 vaccination and masking, is a safe, effective way to help prevent the spread of COVID-19, and help keep schools open for in-person learning. Many people with COVID-19, especially children and teens, don't have symptoms but can still spread the virus, so regular testing helps find people who have the virus before it can spread to others. This is especially important for children who are not yet vaccinated against COVID-19 and those who are not fully vaccinated (first dose and the booster doses) against COVID-19. Finding early who has the virus means that steps can be taken to prevent COVID-19 from spreading and causing an outbreak. Regular testing also means parents or guardians get notified if their child tests positive, allowing them to plan for treatment and take steps to protect the rest of the family from COVID-19.

COVID-19 tests are free, quick, and easy: The tests are free, quick, and easy and will help to prevent COVID spread even if a person does not have symptoms.

Methods of testing: The tests are conducted in laboratories. For the COVID-19 pandemic surge, the US administration has made the lab capacities available to support the additional millions of tests nationwide. The administration has connected COVID-19 testing providers to the American Rescue Plan that have funds for the coronavirus stimulus package.

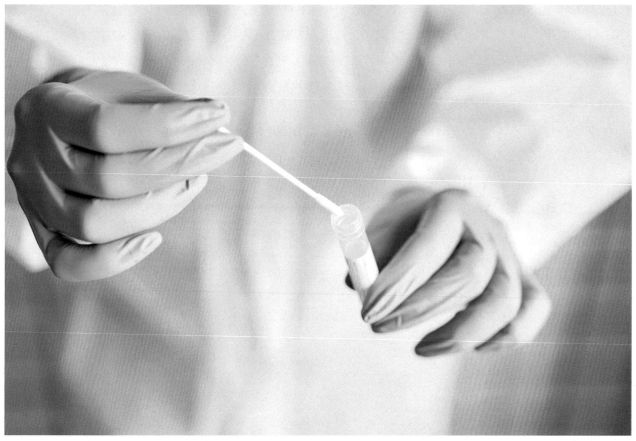

Fig. 2. Sample with a swab for further laboratory analysis (Source: Adobe Stock, 2022).

There are two main types of tests for COVID-19.

Viral tests: Viral tests detect the virus and tell us if there is a current infection. The polymerase chain reaction (PCR) test is the so-called the gold-standard COVID-19 test.

Antibody tests: Antibody tests detect the antibodies make against the viral antigens that tell us if there was a previous infection.

Antibody tests are rapid tests or turn-around fast results and are commonly conducted in non-hospital settings, like nursing homes and university campuses. They are more likely to read out false negatives.

PCR tests are conducted by hospitals and large commercial labs and are the least likely to give false negative results. PCR test relies on finding trace amounts of the virus' genetic material in the test sample. If present, the test copies the viral genome repeatedly, essentially serving as a megaphone that can amplify even a subtle presence of the virus. If there's a very low-level infection present, the PCR test is the most likely test to pick up the presence of the virus.

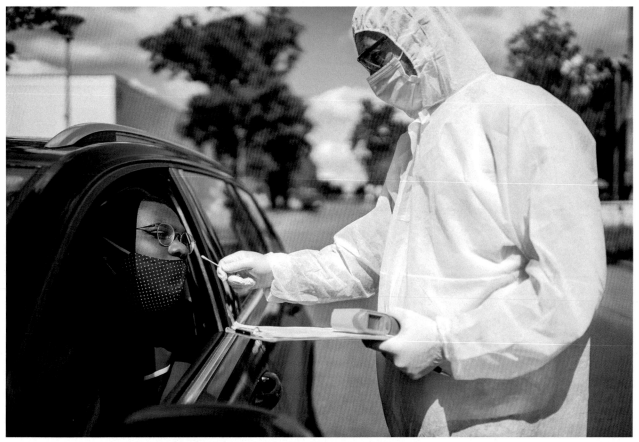

Fig. 3. A healthcare worker administers a COVID-19 swab test at the Boulder County Fairgrounds testing site in Longmont.

There are self-tests as well as tests available at many health centers and pharmacies.

Self-tests: Self-tests are certainly convenient, but there are less accurate for a number of reasons. Spit tests are common for at-home tests but come with some downsides. And people at home (understandably) will have a difficult time shoving a swab into their own nose.

If the self-test result comes out negative, one should be suspicious of that test result. A negative result on one of the faster, less-trustworthy tests warrants a re-test using a gold standard option.

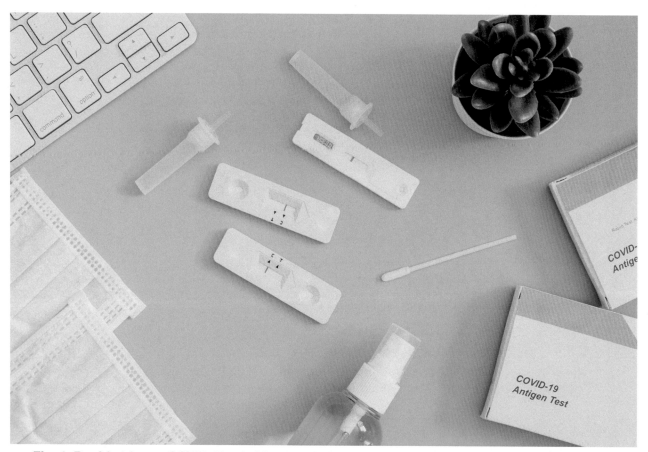

Fig. 4. Rapid at-home COVID-19 test kits are ready to be distributed at the Chelsea Community Connections in Chelsea, Massachusetts (Joseph Prezioso, *AFP*, Getty Images, December 17, 2021).

The Centers for Disease Control and Prevention recommends at-home testing when experiencing COVID-19 symptoms including fever, cough, sore throat, respiratory symptoms, and muscle aches, five days after a potential

COVID-19 exposure or as part of test-to-stay protocols in schools.

US administration provides self-tests to Americans for free ("Fact sheet: The Biden Administration to begin distributing At-home Rapid COVID-19 Tests to Americans for free," statements and releases, January 14, 2022, www. whitehouse.gov).

The spokesperson at the White House said that testing is an important tool to help mitigate the spread of COVID-19. Public health experts and the Centers for Disease Control and Prevention recommend that Americans use at-home tests if they begin to have symptoms, at least five days after coming in close contact with someone who has COVID-19 or is gathering indoors with a group of people who are at risk of severe disease or unvaccinated.

Americans will be able to order their tests online at www.COVIDTests. gov(www.whitehouse.gov;. Statements and Releases, Jan 14, 2022).

The administration has launched a call line to help those unable to access the website to place orders.

The administration is working with national and local community-based organizations to support the nation's hardest-hit and highest-risk communities in requesting tests.

There are now over 20,000 free testing sites across the nation, including four times as many pharmacies participating in the federal pharmacy free testing program as there were in January 2021, as well as federal surge free testing sites, with more free testing sites opening each week.

Millions of free, at-home COVID-19 tests have been delivered to thousands of community health centers and rural health clinics to distribute to their patients, with more delivered each week.

The US administration provided schools with $10 billion in American Rescue Plan (ARP) funding to get tests to K12 school districts. In addition, the administration provided $6 billion in ARP funding to cover free testing for uninsured individuals and support testing in correctional facilities, shelters for people experiencing homelessness, and mental health facilities.

ABC News reached out to all 13 testing companies that have FDA authorization for at-home test kits. In interviews with seven, including five of the largest producers, the testing companies said they were each producing anywhere from a few million to 200 million tests per month.

In this photo illustration, Abbott's at-home COVID-19 rapid test kits are seen on display in Orlando.

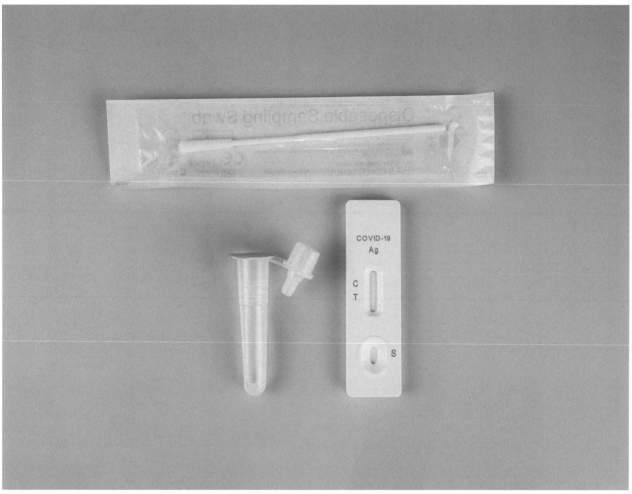

Fig. 5. COVID-19 antigen self-test kit (Paul Hennessy, LightRocket, Getty Images [2022], abbott.com).

The BinaxNOW COVID-19 self-test card is identical to the professional-use test card, used since August 2020 and is the most studied and widely available rapid antigen test and is now available as a self-test (www.abbott.com/BinaxNOW-Tests, accessed on February 21, 2022).

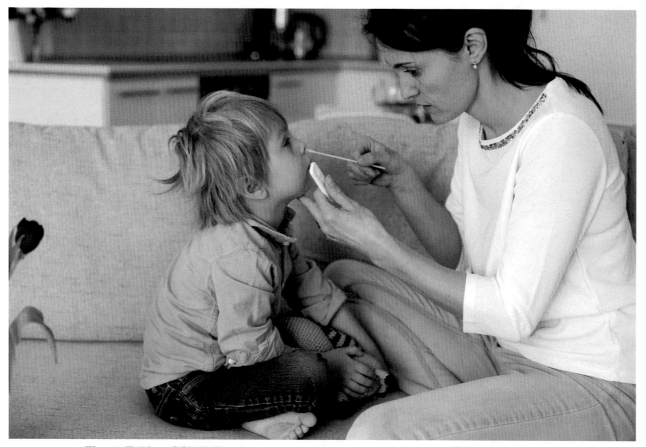

Fig. 6. Taking COVID Testing to a new level (www.abbott.com/BinaxNOW-Tests).

You can now access BinaxNOW test in two ways, at your local retailer over the counter self-test or get it from your healthcare professional. This combination will help attack the pandemic on critical fronts—speed, simplicity, affordability, access, and reliability. *For serial testing, the BinaxNOW COVID-19 Antigen Self-Test should be performed twice over 3 days, at least 24 hours (and no more than 48 hours) apart. For symptomatic use, a single test can be used.*

The BinaxNOW COVID-19 test has a shelf life of 12 months (Food and Drug Administration, www.fda.gov, USA, 2022).

Private insurance companies are required to pay for up to 8 over-the-counter, at-home COVID tests per month, per member (according to a press release by the Medicare & Medicaid Services, USA, January 15, 2022). The typical cost for a two-pack of tests is $24. It could cost Americans almost $100 per month. If you have private health insurance, you should be eligible for reimbursement after you buy an at-home COVID test.

Community-based testing: Testing for SARS-CoV-2 was conducted to evaluate the cost effectiveness and to determine point prevalence in a rural community. The test kits were obtained through Exact Sciences Laboratories, LLC, and Madison, Wisconsin, USA, which partnered with the state of Wisconsin to increase testing capacity and provide testing supplies, laboratory services, and results to any health care provider without cost. The testing procedure used was the real-time reverse transcriptase polymerase chain reaction (RT-PCR) for N gene detection. Collection supplies were used for nasal (anterior nares) collection, including a synthetic-tipped swab on a plastic shaft and RNase-free normal saline transport media.

Samples were stored in a biohazard bag and temperature controlled from the time of collection until shipment by courier for processing the evening of the sample collection. Laboratory processing included extraction of viral RNA from specimens followed by 1-step reverse transcription and PCR amplification with primer and probe sets specific to regions of the SARS-CoV-2 RNA genome (US Food and Drug Administration, accelerated emergency use authorization [EUA]). SARS-CoV-2 (E, N, and RdRP genes) were detected at the Exact Sciences Laboratory. The results showed 1 positive out of 36 high-risk asymptomatic people, and 5 positives in 128 symptomatic patients, confirming the low prevalence of COVID-19 in our area.

Community-based testing sites: The community-based testing sites (CBTS) program were developed by the Federal Emergency Management Agency (FEMA, www.fema.gov, accessed on February 21, 2022) in collaboration with US Health and Human Services (HHS, www.hhs.gov, accessed on February 21, 2022) for states, local public health agencies, healthcare systems, and commercial partners as they work together to stop the spread of COVID-19 in their communities. They released new vaccine and testing mandates.

The task force also prepared and distributed best practices for nasal self-swabbing to collect samples for COVID-19 testing, resulting in a reduction in the amount of required personal protective equipment.

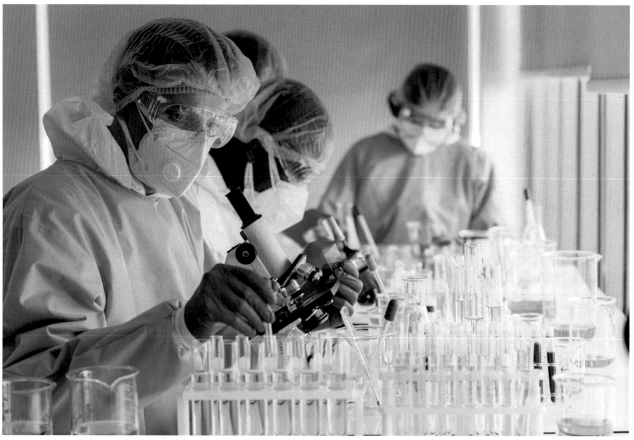

Fig. 7. Arizona's largest laboratory for COVID-19 test operation (www.hhs.gov., USA, 2021).

Health centers: Health centers are an important component of the national response to the COVID-19 pandemic. Health centers, such as local pharmacies, Walmart pharmacies, CVS Health, Rite Aid, Walgreens, etc., are conducting COVID-19 testing and screening. Health centers provide COVID-19 testing services to individuals who meet the criteria for COVID-19 testing regardless of their ability to pay. Check your local health department and local news for additional testing sites in your area. COVID-19 tests are available to everyone in the US, including the uninsured at health centers and select pharmacies nationwide. Additional testing sites may be available in your area. Contact your healthcare provider or your state or local public health department for more information (www.hhs.gov.USA, 2021).

Which test is the best? There are several different types of tests for COVID-19 available in the market today.

At-home COVID-19 tests allow you to know your COVID status, whether you've developed symptoms of the virus or recently had close contact with someone who is infected. While at-home COVID-19 tests are now available to the general public at pharmacies, larger retailers, and even grocery stores and online, they often fly off shelves as soon as they're stocked. If you can find one, it's a good idea to grab it. "It makes sense to have a kit on-hand so it's there if needed," Dr. Amesh A. Adalja, a senior scholar at the Johns Hopkins Center for Health Security, tells *Yahoo Life* (www.yahoo.com, January 17, 2022).

List of at-home COVID tests: With that in mind, we tracked down popular at-home COVID-19 tests that are still in stock. Here's where you can find them (www.yahoo.com, January 17, 2022)

BinaxNow: This popular at-home kit involves taking a nasal swab and waiting 15 minutes for your result. It is available at Walmart, CVS, Amazon, and other stores.

QuickVue: This test kit has you take a nasal swab, put it in a solution, dip it in a test strip and then wait for your results. It is available at so many stores.

On/Go: This kit involves taking a nasal swab, putting it in a solution, squeezing a few drops of the solution into a test kit, and waiting for your results. There's an app to guide you through the whole process. It is available at drug and grocery stores.

FlowFlex: This test was recently authorized by the FDA. It involves swabbing your nose, sticking it in a special solution, and analyzing the solution in a test kit. It is available at CVS, Target, and other stores.

iHealth Rapid Antigen Test: This Amazon bestselling test kit has you take a nasal swab, dip it in a solution, add a few drops of the solution to the test kit, and wait for your results.

These tests have been granted an emergency use authorization (EUA) by the Food and Drug Administration (FDA) during public health emergencies, such as this COVID-19 pandemic.

It is different from full FDA approval, which typically comes only after a longer period of time has passed and more data is collected.

The company (Abbott) claims that MinaxNOW detects 84.6 percent of positive COVID-19 cases and 98.5 percent of negative cases.

The QuickVue At-Home COVID-19 test is another antigen test authorized as EUA. The test kit contains self-collected anterior nasal (nares) swabs from individuals ages 14 and older or individuals ages 8 and older with swabs collected by an adult. The test is authorized for individuals suspected of COVID-19 by their healthcare provider within the first six days of symptom onset. "The FDA continues to prioritize the availability of more at-home testing options in response to the pandemic," said Jeff Shuren, M.D., J.D., director of the FDA's Center for Devices and Radiological Health. "The QuickVue At-Home COVID-19 Test is another example of the FDA working with test developers to bring important diagnostics to the public."

Flow*flex* COVID-19 home test (product of the ACON Laboratories), an over-the-counter (OTC) COVID-19 antigen test adds to the growing list of tests that can be used at home without a prescription. This action highlights our continued commitment to increasing the availability of appropriately accurate and reliable OTC tests to meet public health needs and increase access to testing for consumers. By years end, the manufacturer plans to produce more than 100 million tests per month, and this number will rise to 200 million per month by February 2022. (www.fda.gov., USA, 2022).

We have mentioned just a few OTC at-home tests, but there are many more, and the FDA considers it a high priority and continues to prioritize it as a public health importance.

Other than home testing, there are COVID-19 tests performed by hospitals and healthcare professionals.

Tests performed by health providers (not at-home tests)

Clip COVID Test: The nasal swab specimens are collected by the healthcare provider. Emergency use of this test is limited to authorized laboratories. This test is authorized for use at the point of care (POC) (i.e., in-patient care settings operating under a CLIA Certificate of Waiver, Certificate of Compliance, or Certificate of Accreditation) (www.fda.gov., USA, 2022).

SalivirDetect test: The SalivirDetect test is authorized for use with saliva specimens collected in the presence of a trained observer (adult trained on how to collect saliva samples) from individuals who are either suspected of COVID-19 by their healthcare provider or from individuals without symptoms or other epidemiological reasons to suspect COVID-19 using supervised or unsupervised specimen collection. SalivirDetect is a quantitative reverse transcription polymerase chain reaction method applied to crude saliva samples with no need for RNA isolation (www.fda.gov., USA, 2022).

In summary, unprecedented progress has been made in testing for COVID-19 and the novel ways of diagnosing COVID-19 infections are being searched by scientists. Every effort by governments, industries, and the public all around the world is in force to stop the spread of the COVID-19 pandemic.

CHAPTER 14

PILLS TO TREAT SARS-COV-2

On December 22, 2021, Federal Drug Administration (FDA), USA, gave approval as an emergency authorization for an antiviral pill for COVID-19 to the Pfizer Pharmaceutical Co. (www.pfizer.com) which developed and produced an antiviral pill. It was named Paxlovid.

Paxlovid is the first-ever at-home COVID-19 medication that received FDA (www.fda.gov., USA, 2021) approval as an emergency authorization as an antiviral pill for COVID-19.

According to the press release statement of Dr. Patrizia Cavazzoni, the director of the Center for Drug Evaluation and Research (CDER) at the U.S. Food and Drug Administration, "This authorization provides a new tool to combat COVID-19 at a crucial time in the pandemic as new variants emerge and promises to make antiviral treatment more accessible to patients who are at high risk for progression to severe COVID-19."

On December 23, 2021, the FDA authorized another antiviral pill Molnupiravir, manufactured by Merck Pharmaceutical Co. (www.merck.com), for the treatment of mild to moderate COVID-19 in people ages 18 years and older who are at increased risk for severe illness.

Early distributions of antiviral pills are urgently needed in order to curve the rise in infections and prevent progress to severe illness.

What is a pill? A pill is a small pellet or tablet of medicine, often coated, and taken by swallowing whole or by chewing.

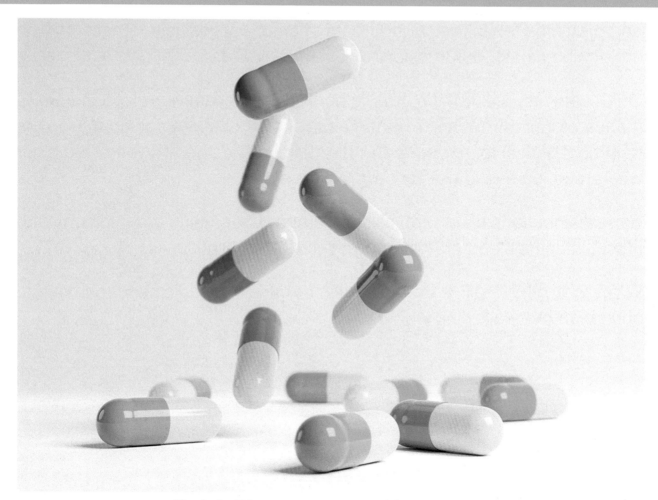

Fig. 1. A pill is a small pellet (www.bing.com**, 2022)**

Oral antiviral medications for COVID-19 treatment: The oral antiviral medications Paxlovid and Molnupiravir have been shown to lower the risk of hospitalization and death in people who are at increased risk of severe COVID-19 illness (www.health.harvard.edu, 2021, cited, December 22, 2021).

1. **Paxlovid as an oral pill for COVID-19 treatment:** Paxlovid as an oral pill is administered as 3 tablets; 2 tablets of Nirmatrelvir and 1 tablet of Ritonavir. The tablets are co-packed as Paxlovid pill.

The 3 tablets are taken together orally twice daily.

Paxlovid is available by prescription only and should be initiated as soon as possible after a diagnosis of COVID-19 and within five days of symptom onset. It has been authorized for the treatment of mild-to-moderate COVID-19 in people ages 12 and older who are at increased risk for severe illness including hospitalization or death.

The chemical structures of the active ingredients:

Chemical name of nirmatrelvir

(1R,2S,5S)-N-((1S)-1-Cyano-2-((3S)-2-   oxopyrrolidin-3-yl)ethyl)-3-((2S)-3,3-dimethyl-2-(2,2,2-trifluoroacetamido)butanoyl)-6,6-dimethyl-3-azabicyclo[3.1.0]hexane-2-carboxamide]

Molecular Formula of Nirmatrelvir: $C_{23}H_{32}F_3N_5O_4$
Molecular weight of Nirmatrelvir: 499.5g/mol
Chemical name of ritonavir

10-Hydroxy-2-methyl-5-(1-methylethyl)-1- [2-(1 methylethyl)-4- thiazolyl]-3,6-dioxo-8,11-bis(phenylmethyl)-2,4,7,12- tetraazatridecan-13-oic acid, 5-thiazolylmethyl ester, [5S-(5R*,8R*,10R*,11R*)].

Molecular formula of ritonavir, $C_{37}H_{48}N_6O_5S_2$
Molecular weight of ritonavir, 720.95 g/mol
Molecular structure of ritonavir (https://pubchem.ncbi.nlm.nih.gov. 1-28-22):

Mechanism of action (MOA) of Paxlovid: Nirmatrelvir, the constituent of Paxlovid, is a protease inhibitor of SARS-CoV-2 and prevents viral replication by blocking the protease from processing the viral polyproteins. Hence, Nirmatrelvir is a potent inhibitor of COVID-19 and its variants including the Omicron variant and prevents replication of the virus.

Treatment studies on Paxlovid: Paxlovid is a prescription medicine. After a positive COVID-19 test and within 5 days of symptom onset, it can be prescribed by the health official.

Drug development, clinical trials, and EPIC-HR: Clinical pharmacology studies during drug development are carried out in three phases.

Phase 1: Phase 1 clinical trial begins after a biopharmaceutical company has filed its Investigational New Drug application (IND) with the U.S. Food and Drug Administration (FDA). Phase 1 studies evaluate pharmacokinetics (PK) and pharmacodynamics (PD) of the drug in humans.

PK profiles explain what the body does to the drug (absorption, distribution, metabolism, and excretion).

PD profiles explain what the drug does to the body.

PK and PD profiles of the drug are influenced by the physicochemical properties of the drug, product/formulation, administration route, patient's intrinsic and extrinsic factors (e.g., organ dysfunction, diseases, concomitant medications, food, etc.). These studies include initial single-dose studies, dose escalation, and short-term repeated-dose studies.

Phase 2: Phase 2 studies explore therapeutic parameters. These are small-scale trials to evaluate a drug's preliminary efficacy and side-effect profile in 100 to 250 patients. Additional safety and clinical pharmacology studies are also included in this category.

Phase 3: Phase 3 is therapeutic confirmatory trials. These are large-scale clinical trials for safety and efficacy in large patient populations. While phase 3 studies are in progress, preparations are made for submitting the biologics license application (BLA) or the new drug application (NDA). BLAs are reviewed by the FDA's Center for Biologics Evaluation and Research (CBER). NDAs are reviewed by the Center for Drug Evaluation and Research (CDER).

Development phases of Paxlovid drug: Paxlovid has passed phase 1, and the data confirmed the potential of Paxlovid as a broad coronavirus antiviral therapeutic (www.fda.gov. 2021). It is now in the phase 2/3 stage.

PAXLOVID has passed Phase 1. It is now in Phase 2/3 stage. Patients received Paxlovid

or placebo orally every 12 hours for 5 days. The phase 2/3 EPIC-HR (evaluation of protease inhibition for COVID-19 in high-risk patients) study safety data showed that Paxlovid significantly reduced hospitalization and death. The phase 2/3 clinical trial included about 1,200 adults from the United States and around the world who had enrolled in the clinical trial. In the overall study population through day 28, no deaths were reported in patients who received Paxlovid as compared to 10 (1.6%) deaths in patients who received placebo. (www.pfizer.com/news/press-release, November 5, 2021).

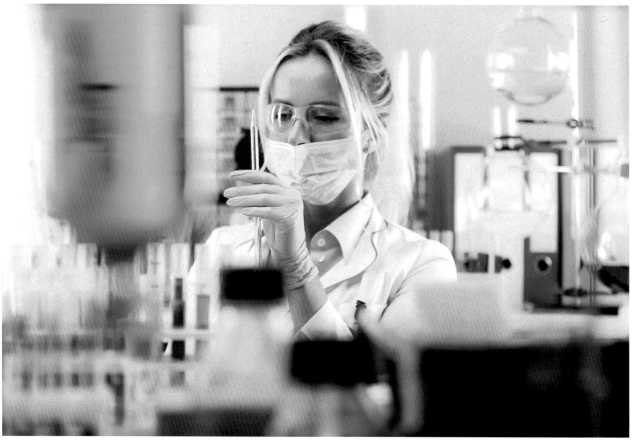

Fig. 2. Clinical studies on Paxlovid as a potential broad coronavirus antiviral oral pill (News release, www.pfizer.com, November 5, 2021).

The Merck Pharmaceutical Co. (www.merck.com), developed an oral pill "Molnupiravir", for the treatment of mild to moderate COVID-19 in people ages 18 years and older who are at increased risk for severe illness.

Merck CEO and President Rob Davis shared the news about the investigational COVID-19 medicine. He stated, "We have a long legacy of research in infectious diseases, we recognized our responsibility to mobilize our scientific expertise and experience to help address this extraordinary global health crisis—but we also recognized the importance of taking care of our people and our communities. In this oral history, our leaders, colleagues and key partners share in their own words how Merck and the world at large were transformed by COVID-19. The COVID-19 pandemic continues to be an unrivaled scientific and global health challenge. We have supported COVID-19 vaccination, diagnosis, and treatment, focused on physical, mental, social, and financial well-being and provided resources to both improve our virtual working environment and help with unique work-life integration challenges".

2. The oral pill Molnupiravir for the treatment of COVID-19:
Chemical name: Molnupiravir
Manufacturer of Molnupiravir: Merck and Ridqeback (www.merck.com)
Molecular structure:

Mechanism of action (MOA) of Molnupiravir: Molnupiravir inhibits the replication of certain RNA viruses including COVID-19. Molnupiravir has demonstrated *in vitro* activity against severe acute respiratory syndrome coronavirus 2 (SARS-CoV-2) in human airway epithelial cell cultures. Prophylactic and therapeutic administration of molnupiravir to mice infected with severe acute respiratory syndrome coronavirus (SARS-CoV) or Middle East respiratory syndrome coronavirus (MERS-CoV) improved pulmonary function and reduced virus titer and body weight loss. In the ferret model of influenza, treatment of pandemic influenza A virus with molnupiravir resulted in reduced viral shedding and inflammatory cellular infiltrates in nasal lavages, with a normal humoral antiviral response.

Clinical Studies on Molnupiravir as an antiviral medication: Early treatment with molnupiravir reduced the risk of hospitalization or death in at-risk, unvaccinated adults with Covid-19. (Funded by Merck Sharp and Dohme; MOVe-OUT ClinicalTrials.gov number, NCT04575597.)

Molnupiravir for oral treatment of COVID-19 in hospitalized patients:

Official title: A phase 2/3 randomized, placebo-controlled, double-blind clinical study of hospitalized adults with COVID-19.

Estimated enrollment: 1,850 participants, randomized
Oral dose of Molnupiravir administered: Variable in milligrams
Intervention model: Parallel assignment
Masking: Double (participants, investigator)
Primary purpose: Treatment

Molnupiravir for oral treatment of COVID-19 in non-hospitalized patients: Molnupiravir (MK-4482) is an oral, small-molecule antiviral prodrug that is active against severe acute respiratory syndrome coronavirus 2 (SARS_CoV-2).

A phase 3, double-blind, randomized, placebo-controlled trial evaluated the efficacy and safety of treatment with molnupiravir started within 5 days after the onset of signs or symptoms in non-hospitalized, unvaccinated adults with mild-to-moderate, laboratory-confirmed Covid-19 and at least one risk factor for severe Covid-19 illness.

Enrollment: 1,433 participants, randomized—716 received Molnupiravir and 717 received placebo. With the exception of an imbalance in sex, baseline characteristics were similar in the two groups.

Oral dose of Molnupiravir administered: 800 mg twice daily for 5 days or placebo
Intervention model: Parallel assignment
Masking: Double (participants, investigator)
Primary purpose: Treatment.

The primary efficacy endpoint was the incidence of hospitalization or death on day 29; the incidence of adverse events was the primary safety endpoint.

Results: The superiority of molnupiravir was demonstrated at the interim analysis; the risk of hospitalization for any cause or death through day 29 was lower with molnupiravir (28 of 385 participants [7.3%]) than with placebo (53 of 377 [14.1%]) (difference, −6.8 percentage points; 95% confidence interval, −11.3 to −2.4; P=0.001). In the analysis of all participants who had undergone randomization, the percentage of participants who were hospitalized or died through day 29 was lower in the molnupiravir group than in the placebo group (6.8% [48 of 709] vs. 9.7% [68 of 699]; difference, −3.0 percentage points; 95% confidence interval, −5.9 to −0.1).

Results of subgroup analyses were largely consistent with these overall results; in some subgroups, such as patients with evidence of previous SARS-CoV-2 infection, those with low baseline viral load, and those with diabetes, the point estimate for the difference favored placebo. One death was reported in the molnupiravir group and 9 were reported in the placebo group through day 29. Adverse events were reported in 216 of 710 participants (30.4%) in the molnupiravir group and 231 of 701 (33.0%) in the placebo group.

Conclusions: Early treatment with molnupiravir reduced the risk of hospitalization or death in at-risk, unvaccinated adults with COVID-19.

Molnupiravir has been shown to be safe and well tolerated in the first-in-human Phase 1 trial in healthy volunteers. Side effects of molnupiravir include diarrhea, nausea, and dizziness. The drug is not recommended for use during pregnancy.

Molnupiravir is also known as EIDD-2801/MK-4482). It is a prodrug of the active antiviral ribonucleoside analog β-D-N4-Hydroxycytidine (NHC; EIDD-1931), which has demonstrated the potential to treat infections caused by multiple RNA viruses, including highly pathogenic coronaviruses and influenza viruses, and encephalitic alphaviruses such as Venezuelan, Eastern, and Western equine encephalitis viruses, in nonclinical models.

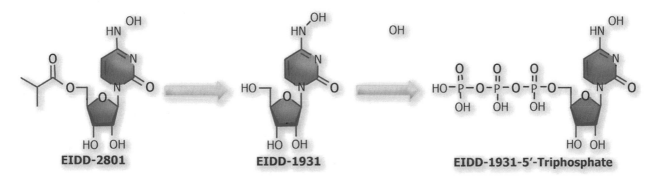

Fig. 3. Structures of Molnupiravir; prodrug to drug. EIDD-1931 (drug name) is chemically N4-Hydroxycitidine.

Molnupiravir is quickly cleaved in plasma to EIDD-1931, which after distribution into various tissues, is converted to its corresponding 5′-triphosphate by host kinases.

EIDD-1931 5′-triphosphate is a competitive alternative substrate for the virally encoded RNA-dependent RNA polymerase, and upon incorporation into nascent chain viral RNA, it induces an antiviral effect via viral error catastrophe, a concept that is predicated on increasing the viral mutation rate beyond a biologically tolerable threshold, resulting in impairment of viral fitness and leading to viral extinction.

3. Antidepressant pills that have shown promise for treating COVID-19:
A large study published in Lancet Global Health in October 2021 found that the antidepressant fluvoxamine (Luvox), which may be taken by mouth at home, significantly reduces the risk of hospitalization in some COVID-19 patients at serious risk for severe illness (www.bing.com/news, 2022).

Antidepressant fluvoxamine is a selective serotonin reuptake inhibitor (SSRI) and a σ-1 receptor (S1R) agonist. There are several potential mechanisms for fluvoxamine in the treatment of COVID-19 illness, including anti-inflammatory and possible antiviral effects. A small placebo-controlled, randomized trial has raised the possibility that fluvoxamine might reduce the risk of clinical deterioration in outpatients with COVID-19, suggesting the need for larger randomized, placebo-controlled studies.

4. More drugs are on the way for treating COVID-19: "Viruses are wily creatures, and you've got to stay ahead of them," said Dr. Anthony Fauci, the government's top infectious disease expert. "I think it would be naïve to think that if you get one or two good drugs, you don't need any more—not when you have a virus that has already killed 760,000 Americans."

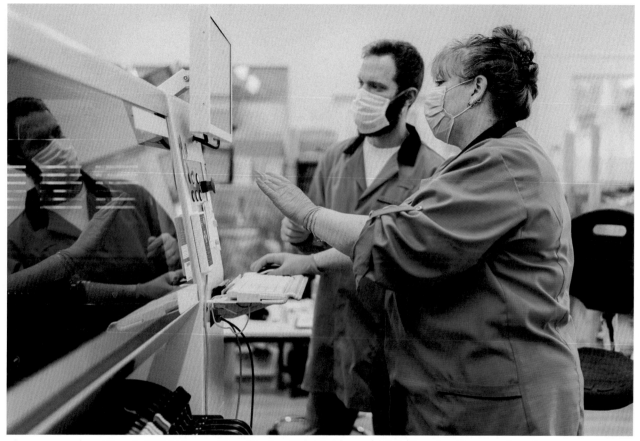

Fig. 4. "Old Drugs May Find a New Purpose: Fighting the Coronavirus"
(***The New York Times,*** **www.nytimes.com, 2021).**

An antiviral drug for COVID-19 that promises to reduce the risk of hospitalization is expected to be authorized by the European Medicines Agency (EMA) this week. It should mark the start of another year of developments around vaccines and treatments against viruses and more potential surges or flare-ups (https://www.msn.com/, January 31, 2022).

CHAPTER 15

EMERGENCE OF VARIANTS OF CORONAVIRUS

The US Department of Health and Human Services (HHS) established a SARS-CoV-2 Interagency Group (SIG) to improve coordination among the Centers for Disease Control and Prevention (CDC), National Institutes of Health (NIH), Food and Drug Administration (FDA), Biomedical Advanced Research and Development Authority (BARDA), and Department of Defense (DoD). This interagency group is focused on the rapid characterization of emerging variants and actively monitors their potential impact on critical SARS-CoV-2 countermeasures, including vaccines, therapeutics, and diagnostics.

Viruses constantly change through mutation, and new variants of a virus are expected to occur. Sometimes new variants emerge and disappear; other times new variants persist. All variants of the virus that cause COVID-19 are being tracked in the United States and globally during this pandemic by the Centers for Disease Control and Prevention (www.cdc.gov, USA, 2021).

CDC continues to monitor all variants circulating within the United States. Viruses continuously evolve as changes in the genetic code (gene mutations) occur during the replication of the genome.

Variant: A variant with one or more mutations becomes a new variant.

Mutation: A mutation is a change in a DNA sequence. Mutations can result from DNA copying mistakes made during cell division or exposure to ionizing radiation or exposure to chemicals called mutagens.

Germline mutations occur in the eggs and sperm and can be passed on to offspring, while somatic mutations occur in body cells and are not passed on.

Mutation is really a simple process of a mistake made in a DNA sequence as it is being copied. DNA copying is not perfect, and it results in changes in DNA and that leads to evolution as well as to genetic diseases.

But mutation can also be induced by things like radiation or carcinogens in a way that can increase the risk of cancers or birth defects. But it's pretty simple; it's basically an induced misspelling of the DNA sequence. That's a mutation (Francis S. Collins, 2021). Mutation is explained diagrammatically in fig.1.

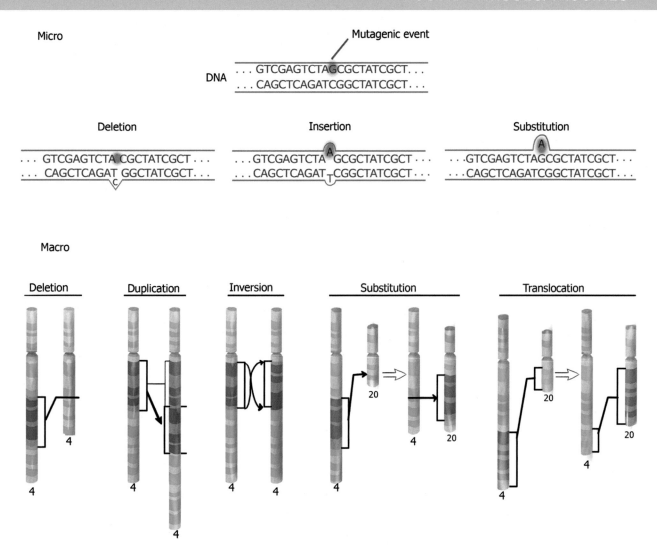

Fig. 1. Mutation: It is a change in a DNA sequence resulting from the copying of DNA during cell division (https://www.genome.gov, 2021).

As the SARS-CoV-2 virus circulates worldwide, it is making copies of itself and replicating and giving rise to the chances of mutations and making new variants.

DNA Sequence: In the previous chapter, we discussed DNA vaccines and the structure of DNA briefly. Now we will look into the structure of DNA with regard to mutations and variants.

DNA is the genetic material and has the unique double-helical shape. DNA analysis identifies variations (mutations) in genes, chromosomes, or proteins that cause genetic disorders. Many inherited diseases occur due to genetic disorders.

Genetic disorders:

> single-gene inheritance
> multifactorial inheritance
> chromosome abnormalities
> mitochondrial inheritance

Single-gene inheritance disorders: Single gene inheritance is also called Mendelian or monogenetic inheritance. This is due to changes or mutations in the DNA sequence of a single gene. Here are a few examples of Single Gene Inheritance Disorders:

Inheritance of cystic fibrosis (CF): Cystic fibrosis is an inherited disease that affects the secretory glands, the sweat and mucus glands, lungs, livers, pancreas, and sex organs. CF is due to a mutation in the CF gene that encodes cystic fibrosis transmembrane regulator (CFTR) on chromosome 7. The abnormal CFTR protein in patients with CF leads to disruption in chloride channels in the cells.

Every person inherits two CFTR genes, one from each parent. CF is inherited in an autosomal recessive manner; a child who inherits a faulty gene from each parent will have CF. A child who inherits one mutant and one normal gene will be CF carrier. CF carriers usually have no symptoms of CF but can pass the faulty gene on to their children. If each parent has a normal CFTR gene and a faulty CFTR gene, each child has a 25 percent chance of inheriting two normal genes; a 50 percent chance of inheriting one normal gene and one faulty gene; and a 25 percent chance of inheriting two faulty genes (www.medicinenet.com, 2021).

The image shows how CF genes are inherited. There is no cure for CF, but treatments, nutrition and respiratory therapies, medicines, and exercise can improve both the quality of life and lifespan.

Inheritance of sickle-cell disease (SCD): Sickle-cell disease (SCD) is an autosomal-recessive genetic disorder (in which two copies of a defective gene, one from each parent) are necessary to cause the condition). SCD affects approximately 100,000 people in the United States and millions worldwide. In SCD, a single amino acid substitution in the β-globin chain leads to the polymerization of mutant hemoglobin S, impairing erythrocyte rheology and survival. Clinically, erythrocyte abnormalities in SCD manifest in hemolytic anemia.

Inheritance of Marfan syndrome: Marfan syndrome is an autosomal dominant inheritance disorder. Mutations in the fibrillin-1 (*FBN1*) gene cause Marfan syndrome (MFS) and have been associated with a wide range of overlapping phenotypes. It affects connective tissue and adversely impacts multiple organs, including the skeletal system, the ocular system, the cardiovascular system, fascia, skin, and the dural sac. The prevalence is estimated to be between one in 5,000 and one in 10,000 people in all countries and races with similar distributions in both genders

Inheritance of fragile X syndrome (FXS): Fragile X syndrome is a dominant X-chromosome inheritance disorder. The FXS disorder is caused by variants of genes on the X chromosome. In males (who have only one X chromosome), a variant in the only copy of the gene in each cell causes the disorder. In females (who have two X chromosomes), a variant in one of the two copies of the gene in each cell is sufficient to cause the disorder. Females may experience less severe symptoms of the disorder than males. A characteristic of X-linked inheritance is that fathers cannot pass X-linked traits to their sons (no male-to-male transmission).

FXS is caused by the mutations in the *FMR1* gene that makes a protein called FMRP. FMRP is needed for brain development. People with FXS do not make this protein, whereas people with fragile X-associated disorders usually make some of the protein. FXS affects both males and females. However, females often have milder symptoms than males. The exact number of people who have FXS is unknown, but a review of research studies estimated that about 1 in 7,000 males, whereas about 1 in 11,000 females have been diagnosed with FXS (www.cdc.gov, USA, 2021).

Inheritance of hemophilia A and hemophilia B: Hemophilia A & B are inherited X-linked recessive disorders. They are caused by mutations in different genes. Hemophilia A (also known as classic hemophilia or factor

VIII deficiency) and Hemophilia B (also known as Christmas disease or factor IX deficiency), both slow down the blood clotting process and result in excessive bleeding Both have very similar signs and symptoms (www. cdc.gov, USA, 2021).

Y chromosome infertility: Y chromosome infertility is caused by changes in the Y chromosome, one of the sex chromosomes. Genes in these regions are believed to provide instructions for making proteins involved in sperm cell development. A pathogenic variant, USP9Y located in the AZFA region of the Y chromosome can cause Y chromosome infertility. This condition affects the production of sperm; it could be no sperm cells (azoospermia), a few sperms (oligospermia), or abnormally shaped sperm cells (https:// rarediseases.info.nih.gov/diseases, accessed on February 22, 2022).

ABO blood groups: The blood group genes are autosomal inheritance. The *A* and *B* alleles are codominant, and the *O* allele is recessive. In codominance, both alleles are expressed (i.e., neither allele can mask the expression of the other allele). So if an individual inherits allele A from their mother and allele B from their father, they have blood type AB.

There are four common blood groups in the ABO system: O, A, B, and AB. The blood groups are defined by the presence of specific carbohydrate sugars on the surface of red blood cells, N-acetylgalactosamine for the A antigen, and D-galactose for the B antigen. Both of these sugars are built upon the H antigen—if the H antigen is left unmodified, the resulting blood group is O because neither the A nor the B antigen can attach to the red blood cells (https://www.ncbi.nlm.nih.gov., accessed on February 22, 2022).

Individuals will naturally develop antibodies against the ABO antigens they do not have. For example, individuals with blood group A will have anti-B antibodies, and individuals with blood group O will have both anti-A and anti-B. Before a blood transfusion takes place, routine serological testing checks the compatibility of the ABO (and Rh) blood groups. An ABO-incompatible blood transfusion can be fatal, due to the highly immunogenic nature of the A and B antigens, and the corresponding strongly hemolytic antibodies.

Rhesus (Rh) factor is an inherited protein found on the surface of red blood cells. If an individual's blood has the protein, the individual is Rh-positive. If the blood lacks the protein, the individual is Rh-negative.

Rh-positive is the most common blood type. Having an Rh-negative blood type is not an illness and usually does not affect the individual's health. However, it can affect the female individual's pregnancy. The female needs special care if she is Rh negative and her baby is Rh positive (Rh incompatibility). A baby can inherit the Rh factor from either parent. The health care provider will recommend a blood type and Rh factor screening test during her first prenatal visit. This will identify whether your blood cells carry the Rh factor protein.(https://www.mayoclinic.org/, accessed on February 22, 2022).

Over 80 *ABO* alleles have been reported. The common alleles include *A1, A2, B1, O1, O1v,* and *O2* Whereas the *A* and *B* alleles each encode a specific glycosyl-transferring enzyme, the *O* allele appears to have no function. A single-base deletion in the *O* allele means that individuals with blood group

O do not produce either the A or B antigens. Blood type frequencies vary in different racial/ethnic groups. In the US, in Caucasians, the ratio of blood group O, A, B, and AB is 45%, 40%, 11%, and 4% respectively. In Hispanics, the distribution is 57%, 31%, 10%, and 3%; and in Blacks, 50%, 26%, 20%, and 4%.

Multifactorial inheritance: Multifactorial inheritance is caused by genes and other factors that are not genes, such as nutrition, pollution, medicines or illness.

Heritability is a measure of how well differences in people's genes account for differences in their traits. Traits can include characteristics such as height, eye color, and intelligence, as well as disorders like schizophrenia and autism spectrum disorder.

In scientific terms, heritability is a statistical concept (represented as H^2) that describes how much of the variation in a given trait can be attributed to genetic variation. An estimate of the heritability of a trait is specific to one population in one environment, and it can change over time as circumstances change.

$H^2 = VG/VP$; VG = Genetic Values; VP = Phenotypic Values.

Broad-sense heritability, H^2 captures the proportion of phenotypic values due to genetic values. The genetic values include dominance and epistasis.

Epistasis is a phenomenon in genetics in which the effect of a gene mutation is dependent on the presence or absence of mutations in one or more other genes, termed 'modifier genes'. In other words, the effect of the mutation is dependent on the genetic background in which it appears.

Acquired characteristics, by definition, are characteristics that are gained by an organism after birth as a result of external influences or the organism's own activities which change its structure or function and cannot be inherited.

Heritability ranges from zero to one. Heritability close to zero indicates that almost all of the variability in a trait among people is due to environmental factors, with very little influence from genetic differences. Characteristics such as religion, language spoken, and political preference have a heritability of zero because they are not under genetic control. Heritability close to one indicates that almost all of the variability in a trait comes from genetic differences, with very little contribution from environmental factors. Many disorders that are caused by variants (also known as mutations) in single genes, such as phenylketonuria (PKU), have high heritability. Most complex traits in people, such as intelligence and multifactorial diseases, have heritability somewhere in the middle, suggesting that their variability is due to a combination of genetic and environmental factors.

Heritability has historically been estimated from studies of twins. Identical twins have almost no differences in their DNA, while fraternal twins share, on average, 50 percent of their DNA. If a trait appears to be more similar in identical twins than in fraternal twins (when they were raised together in the same environment), genetic factors likely play an important role in determining that trait. By comparing a trait in identical twins versus fraternal twins, researchers can calculate an estimate of its heritability. Heritability does not indicate what proportion of a trait is determined by genes and what proportion is determined by environment. So, a heritability of 0.7 does not mean that a trait is 70% caused by genetic factors; it means that 70% of the variability in the trait in a population is due to genetic differences among people. (www.medlineplus.gov, 2021).

Here are a few examples of multifactorial inheritance:

Birth defects: Viruses and the recent coronavirus pandemic have been shown to be responsible for severe complications during pregnancy; such as miscarriage, fetal growth restriction and congenital anomalies (www.ncbi. nlm.nih.gov, 2021).

Coronary artery disease (CAD): CAD is a multifactorial disease and is increasing in prevalence worldwide. Coronary artery disease is partially explained by genetics and is known to run in families. However, lifestyle and environmental factors, such as diet, contribute to coronary artery disease and heart failure. Hypercholesterolemia and cholesterol metabolic pathways have a key role in CAD pathogenesis (H. Watkins, M. Farrall, 2006).

Diabetes type 2: It is caused by multiple genes (polygenic) in combination with dietary factors, obesity, and pollutants. It is a complex multifactorial disorder. Although complex disorders often cluster in families, they do not have a clear-cut pattern of inheritance. It may be difficult to identify the role of genetics in these disorders, particularly because families often also share environments and may have similar lifestyles. This makes it difficult to determine a person's risk of inheriting or passing on these disorders.

Complex disorders are also difficult to study and treat because the specific factors that cause most of these disorders have not yet been identified.

There are many more multifactorial inheritance that are caused by both genes and other factors, such as Alzheimer disease, arthritis, asthma and allergies, autoimmune disorders, bipolar disorder, multiple sclerosis, osteoporosis, schizophrenia, skin conditions such as psoriasis, moles, and eczema. Researchers continue to look for major contributing genes for many common, complex disorders (www.medlineplus.gov, 2021).

Chromosomal abnormalities: Chromosomal abnormalities are numerical or structural (www.genome.gov, 2021).

Numerical chromosomal abnormality means that an individual is missing one of the chromosomes or has an extra chromosome. Structural abnormalities mean that the chromosomal morphology is altered.

Chromosomes: Chromosomes are thread-like structures located inside the nucleus of animal and plant cells. It is made up of a single molecule of deoxyribonucleic acid (DNA) wrapped in spool-like proteins, called histones. Without such packaging, DNA molecules would be too long to fit inside cells. The term chromosome comes from the Greek words; Chroma (color) and Soma (body), because chromosome is strongly stained by the dyes used in research. It is also crucial that reproductive cells, such as egg and sperm, contain the right number of chromosomes and that those chromosomes have the correct structure. (www.genome.gov, 2021).

Chromosomes have two segments, called "arms," separated by a pinched region known as the centromere. The shorter arm, which is the upper half, is called the p arm. The longer arm, which is the lower half, is called the q arm.

Chromosomes are the structures that hold genes. Genes are the individual instructions that tell our bodies how to develop and function; they govern physical and medical characteristics, such as hair color, blood type and susceptibility to disease.

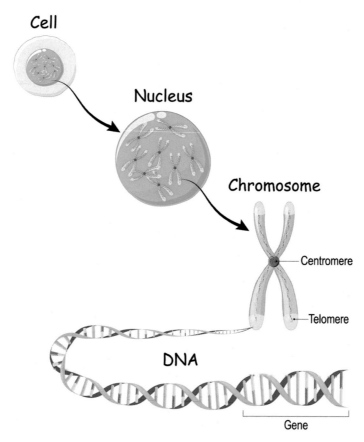

Fig. 2. Chromosome structure (www.genome.gov, 2021).

Humans have 23 pairs of chromosomes, for a total of 46 chromosomes. One set of 23 chromosomes is inherited from the mother (from the egg), and the other set is inherited from the father (sperm). Each parent contributes 22 non-sex chromosomes and one sex chromosome. Females have two X chromosomes in their cells, while males have one X and one Y chromosome. The mother contributes X chromosome, and the father contributes either an X or Y chromosome. Thus, the contribution from the father determines the sex of the baby.

The only human cells that do not contain pairs of chromosomes are reproductive cells, or gametes, which carry just one copy of each chromosome. When two reproductive cells unite, they become a single cell that contains two copies of each chromosome. This cell then divides and its successors divide numerous times, eventually producing a mature individual with a full set of paired chromosomes in virtually all of its cells.

The typical number of chromosomes in a human cell is 46: 23 pairs, holding an estimated total of 20,000 to 25,000 genes. One set of 23 chromosomes is inherited from the biological mother (from the egg), and the other set is inherited from the biological father (from the sperm).

Of the 23 pairs of chromosomes, the first 22 pairs are called "autosomes." The final pair is called the "sex chromosomes." Sex chromosomes determine an individual's sex: females have two X chromosomes (XX), and males have an X and a Y chromosome (XY). The mother and father each contribute one set of 22 autosomes and one sex chromosome.

For a century, scientists studied chromosomes by looking at them under a microscope. In order for chromosomes to be seen this way, they need to be stained. Once stained, the chromosomes look like strings with light and dark "bands," and their picture can be taken. A picture, or chromosome map, of all 46 chromosomes is called a karyotype. The karyotype can help identify abnormalities in the structure or the number of chromosomes.

To help identify chromosomes, the pairs have been numbered from 1 to 22, with the 23rd pair labeled "X" and "Y." In addition, the bands that appear after staining are numbered; the higher the number, the farther that area is from the centromere.

In the past decade, newer techniques have been developed that allow scientists and doctors to screen for chromosomal abnormalities without using a microscope. These newer methods compare the patient's DNA to a normal DNA sample. The comparison can be used to find chromosomal abnormalities where the two samples differ.

There are many types of chromosome abnormalities.

Chromosomal abnormalities can be organized into two basic groups: numerical abnormalities and structural abnormalities.

Numerical chromosome abnormalities: The numerical chromosome abnormalities are known as aneuploidy. They are genetic conditions in which the number of chromosomes in the nucleus of a cell deviates from the diploid number due to an extra or missing chromosome. When an individual is missing one of the chromosomes from a pair, the condition is called monosomy. When an individual has more than two chromosomes instead of a pair, the condition is called trisomy. They are genetic conditions in which the number of chromosomes in the nucleus of a cell deviates from the diploid number due to an extra or missing chromosome. So, instead of the typical 46 chromosomes in each cell of the body, there may be 45 or 47 chromosomes. The electric charge properties of chromosomes could be responsible for the development of these abnormalities.

Examples of numerical abnormalities:

Down syndrome: An individual with Down syndrome has three copies of chromosome 21 rather than two; for that reason, the condition is also known as Trisomy 21. It is marked by mental retardation, learning difficulties, a characteristic facial appearance and poor muscle tone (hypotonia) in infancy.

Turner syndrome: An individual with Turner syndrome lacks a chromosome. In Turner syndrome, a female is born with only one sex chromosome, an X, and is usually shorter than average and unable to have children, among other difficulties.

Patau syndrome: An individual with Patau syndrome has an extra copy of chromosome 13, a medium-length acrocentric chromosome. It is most severe of the viable autosomal trisomies. It results in severe mental deficiency; holopros-encephaly, polydactyly, neural tube defects and heart defects (www.emedicine.medscape.com, updated 2021).

Chromosomal Structural Abnormalities: Structural abnormalities are when a part of a chromosome is missing, or contains an extra part, or is turned upside down.

Structural abnormalities usually occur when there is an error in cell division. There are two kinds of cell division, mitosis and meiosis.

Mitosis results in two cells and it is the way most of the cells that make up our body are made and replaced.

Meiosis takes place in the reproductive organs, resulting in the eggs and sperms. Meiosis results in half of the number of chromosomes, i.e., 23 (in the sperm, or the egg), instead of the normal 46.

Examples of structural abnormalities:

Cri du Chat or cat cry syndrome: It is a genetic syndrome caused by a deletion of #5 chromosome; written as 5p. Since a part of the instructions is missing, it results in the errors in the development of the baby. Babies with Cri du Chat have a small head size, low birth weight, and poor muscle tone. Other health problems can be present; problems with feeding, walking, severe intellectual disability, and other serious organ defects

Pallister Killian syndrome: It is caused by mixture of different chromosomes (mosaicism), some that are have 46 chromosomes with the extra p12 chromosomal material, and some without p12 material. Babies with this syndrome have health problems including seizures, hearing and heart defects. People with Pallister Killian have a shortened lifespan, but may live into their 40s.

Mitochondrial inheritance disorders: Mitochondrial inheritance disorders cause impaired oxidative phosphorylation that affects nearly all cells in the body. Each cell has several hundred mitochondria in its cytoplasm. Mitochondria contain DNA in a single circular chromosome that codes for 13 proteins, various RNAs, and several regulating enzymes. All mitochondria are inherited from the cytoplasm of the egg; thus, mitochondrial DNA comes only from the mother.

Mitochondria are the "energy factory" of our body. Several thousand mitochondria are in nearly every cell in the body. Their job is to process oxygen and convert substances from the foods we eat into energy.

The mitochondrial respiratory chain is the essential final common pathway for aerobic metabolism.

The pathogenic variants in genes coding for the mitochondrial respiratory chain and related proteins are considered to be the primary causes of mitochondrial disorders. Mitochondrial DNA (mtDNA) located within mitochondria, along with the ribosomal and transfer RNAs are involved in the intra-mitochondrial protein synthesis. The remaining respiratory chain polypeptides and proteins essential for the assembly of the respiratory chain, mitochondrial structure, and the maintenance and expression of mtDNA are encoded by the nuclear genome (nDNA) (P. F. Chinnery, 2021).

Examples of Mitochondrial inheritance disorders (https://emedicine. medscape.com, 2021):

Chronic progressive external ophthalmoplegia (CPEO): CPEO is a disorder characterized by slowly progressive paralysis of the extraocular muscles. It is the most frequent manifestation of mitochondrial myopathies. CPEO in association with mutations in mitochondrial DNA (mtDNA) may occur in the absence of any other clinical sign, but it is usually associated with skeletal muscle weakness.

Mitochondrial encephalomyopathy lactic acidosis stroke-like episodes (MELAS): MELAS is acute at the onset, often transient, and occasionally associated with febrile illness. This syndrome is due to point or microdeletion mutations in mitochondrial DNA; as in all diseases with mitochondrial transmission, the disease is inherited via the ovum and hence always from the mother. Mitochondrial DNA is 10 times more prone to mutation than somatic DNA.

Mitochondrial diseases are chronic, genetic, and can affect any part of the body, including the cells of the brain, nerves, muscles, kidneys, heart, liver, eyes, ears or pancreas. Mitochondrial dysfunction can lead to Alzheimer's disease, muscular dystrophy, Lou Gerig's disease, diabetes, and Cancer.

One in 5,000 individuals has a genetic mitochondrial disease. Each year, about 1,000 to 4,000 children in the United States are born with a mitochondrial disease. With the number and type of symptoms and organ systems involved, mitochondrial diseases are often mistaken for other, more common diseases.

CHAPTER 16

EPIDEMIOLOGICAL APPROACHES TO COVID-19 DISEASE SPREAD AND CONTROL

Epidemiology is the study of the distribution and determinants of health-related states or events in specified populations, and the application of this study to the control of health problems. Epidemiology is the foundation of public health because it helps us understand not only who has the disease or disorder, but also why and how it was brought in.

(www.cdc.gov, searched on May 25, 2022).
Epidemiology covers a wide range of issues.
In this chapter, we will cover the following main topics that are related to COVID-19 epidemic:

1. identify the infecting agent

2. track and trace the infecting agent

3. appropriate responses and interventions.

4. educate people on techniques to avoid the transmission of communicable diseases

1. Identify the infecting agent: You can identify the infecting agent from the symptoms it causes. For example, in case of hepatitis A virus (HAV), a communicable disease, patients who are symptomatic, most often present with acute onset fever, malaise, jaundice, hepatomegaly, and abdominal pain. Jaundice is often followed with marked elevated of serum aminotransferases that is greater than 1000 units/L. The test of choice is IgM anti-hepatitis A virus for diagnostic purposes (www.mayoclinic.org)

The detection and identification of the infecting agent/agents for COVID-19 disease are essential for understanding the recent global outbreaks.

SARS-CoV-2 is the infecting agent in COVID-19 outbreaks. Now the emergence of sub-variants; BA.1, BA.1.1, BA.2, and BA.2.12.1 of Omicron, SARS-CoV-2 are rapidly becoming more efficient in transmission and in evading immunity.

The recent COVID-19 outbreak is global. Its symptoms have a wide spectrum; ranging from asymptomatic to critical including mortality. The symptoms were summed up as mild cold (pneumonia), dyspnea, critical respiratory failure to multi-organ failure.

On December 31, 2019, a cluster of cases of pneumonia in people in Huanan seafood wholesale market in China were reported. On January 7, 2020, Chinese health authorities confirmed that a novel Corona virus was the causative agent. The data indicated that person-to-person transmission of CoV was occurring.

2. Track and trace the infecting agent: The patients initial mild symptoms and their progression to pneumonia on day 9 of illness confirmed the identification, diagnosis and clinical course of COVID-19.

Epidemiologic data indicated that a total of 9,976 cases were reported in at least 21 countries as of January 30, 2020, including the first confirmed case of CoV infection in the United States. The close coordination between clinicians and public health authorities at the local, state, and federal levels, and the rapid dissemination of clinical information led to the care of patients with this emerging infection.

3. Appropriate responses and interventions: To control the spread of COVID-19 in U.S.A., the Center for Disease Control and Prevention assesses the community levels and recommends the steps to take to prevent the spread. The levels; low, medium, or high are determined by hospital bed utilization, hospital admissions, and total number of COVID-19 cases in a community (www.cdc.gov, USA, 2021).

Face masks: Wearing a face mask has become essential in order to protect oneself and others from getting or spreading COVID-19. Mandates for mask use during COVID-19 pandemic have been issued by local and federal agencies and updated from time to time. Masks reduce the transmission of respiratory droplets and thus the spread of virus. Mask is an important tool to decrease community transmission and protect health care system capacity during the highly infectious Delta and Omicron surge. Masking is an important layer of protection along with the vaccinations, testing and ventilation, to keep schools and indoor settings safe. Masks are a part of a comprehensive strategy of measures to decrease transmission and protect lives; they are not sufficient alone to provide an adequate protection against COVID-19.

The demand for face masks around the world skyrocketed and many types evolved depending upon the materials, effectiveness and costs. Hence, there are many high-quality masks available that could give adequate protection and are recommended by the experts.

The data are available about almost all the countries in the world which require public mask usage or recommend masks in public to help contain COVID-19 ("Masks for All," 2021, updated).

The worldwide consumption of face masks has been estimated as 129 billion each month since the start of the COVID-19 pandemic.

At the onset of COVID-19, there was severe scarcity in personal protective equipment (PPE). The industries, scientists and governments faced tremendous pressure to meet the demand of face masks for health care workers and the public. It became mandatory in many countries to wear masks for protection.

A variety of face masks have been developed that can meet the basic requirements; high filtration capacity, appropriate type of fiber for providing convenience, and performance.

Face masks: Face masks are devices that cover the nose and mouth so that air gets filtered upon breathing. These are made of fabrics; cotton, flannel, synthetic fabrics, etc. They provide physical barrier against respiratory droplets, and could keep the viruses including COVID-19 out.

Different types of face masks are being manufactured and are available (Amazon.com):

Single-use face masks: They are intended for one time use, and then disposed of. They are made of polypropylene. These are most prevalent among the public and health care workers. These are of high filtration capacity (meaning these do not let viruses and other microorganisms of different sizes to get in), lightweight and affordable. Because of these qualities, they are being mass produced in over 170 countries.

The face masks production takes place all over the world; there are multiple variations in the materials and technologies of production.

According to National Institute for Occupational Safety and Health (NIOSH), the facepiece respirators are further classified according to their filtration percentage and oil resistance:

Table 1: NIOSH-approved Filtering Facepiece Respirator Classification

Type of filtering facepiece	Definition
N	Non-oil-resistant
N95	95% of airborne particulates filters, as small as 300nm
R	Resistant to oil
P	Proof to oil

N95 masks offer protection against SARS-CoV-2 virus.

Surgical N95 respirators are a subset of N95 respirators protect against airborne as well as fluid hazards used by Health care professionals. These respirators are approved by NIOSH and authorized by the FDA, USA. (CDC. gov, 2020).

Types of masks and respirators available in markets approved by U.S. and European standards (www.ncbi.nlm.gov, accessed on January 10, 2022. Doi: 10.1021/acs.chas.1c00016) (fig. 1).

Most common types of respirators, *cloth mask*, is the simplest option used by many people with minimum protection against microscopic particles but capable of filtering large dust-type particles. *Surgical mask,* usually one side is light blue, and the other side remains white, mostly used by healthcare providers. Additionally, it is loosely fitted over the mouth and nose, is fluid-resistant, and mostly prevents entry by large droplets. Respirators following US standards *N95*, these respirators filter out at least 95% of airborne particulates and aerosols as small as 300 nm. *N100*: These respirators filter at least 99.97% of airborne particulates and aerosols as small as 300 nm. *P100*: These respirators remove at least 99.97% of airborne particulates and aerosols. *R95*: These respirators filter (at least 95%) oil- and non-oil-based particles with increased durability. Respirators following European standards: *FFP1*: Filters out 80% of 300 nm particles. *FFP2*: A tightly fitted device reduces exposure to airborne particles with a filtering efficiency of greater than or equal to 94%. *FFP3*: Similar to the N100-type respirator with slightly lower filtration efficiency.

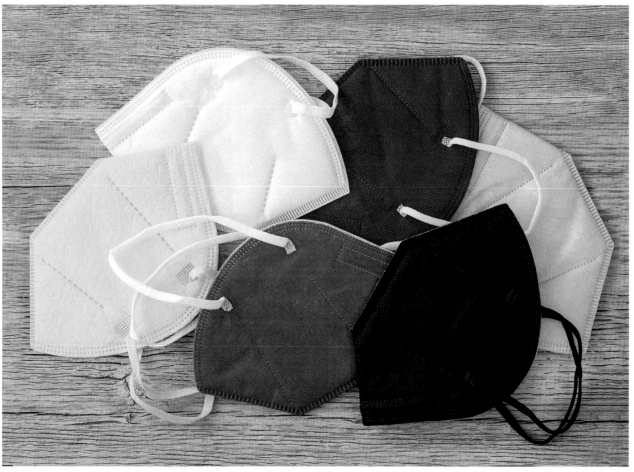

Fig. 1. KN95 masks, 30 packs colorful, individually wrapped KN95 face mask (available at www.amazon.com, searched on June 4, 2022).

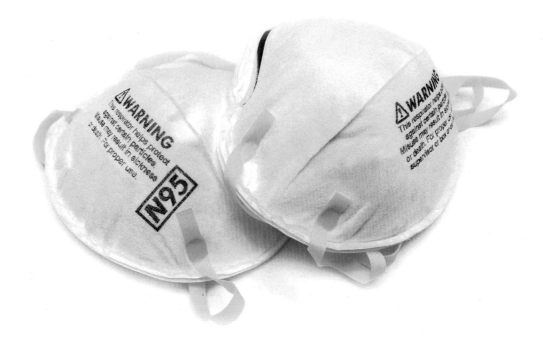

Fig. 2. A stock image of a N95 respirator mask made by 3M. The company makes 95 million N95 masks at two US facilities but check the label—3M also produces masks overseas. *Getty Images*

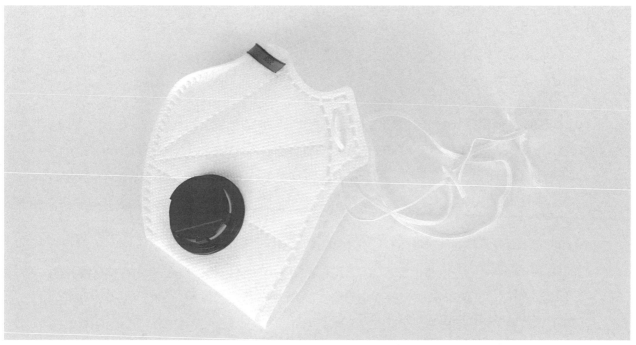

Fig. 3. Flat-fold STS-F100 N95 NIOSH-approved respirator, a box of 50 for $54.00 (https://shop.projectn95.org/, May 30, 2022).

The Project N95 Marketplace is your trusted source for vetted personal protective equipment (PPE) and COVID-19 test kits from verified suppliers.

4. Educating people on techniques to avoid the transmission of communicable diseases:

Education is very important part to take hold of communicable diseases in the context of COVID-19 and its variants. Here are a few protective measures that everybody should know and practice during this global pandemic.

    1. Hand hygiene, discussed earlier in other chapters

2. Physical distancing, discussed earlier in other chapters

3. Wearing masks, discussed in great length in this chapter under item 3.

4. Listening to the infection control experts and the current news about new variants. The health departments provide advice and information about the infection, prevention, and control to the communities.

The emergence of the Omicron variant was revealed in 2020 and showed that it has greater transmissibility as compared to Delta, Alfa, and other previous variants. As discussed in previous chapters, viruses evolve and change constantly. Scientists monitor the viruses globally, as well as in the USA, and study their characteristics; genetics, phenotypes, transmissibility, ability to cause diseases, and vaccine-resistant compared to the original strains.

As more cases of new variants of Omicron emerge around the world, experts say it is likely that variants had been circulating for some time. The World Health Organization (WHO) said that at least 23 countries have now reported cases of Omicron, and we expect that number to grow (www.cnbc.com/2021/12/02).

The origin of the Omicron variant is still unknown. This is due to the limited DNA sequencing data and surveillance. "Our surveillance system in the global world is not perfect yet," Dr. Abdou Salam Gueye, regional emergency director in WHO's Africa office, told CNBC Thursday during a press briefing. When we detect a variant or virus, usually we're going to detect it weeks after it was in circulation.

The highly transmissible Omicron variant emerged with unusual mutations. The evolutionary virologists described it as very different from its known genetic ancestors.

The WHO officials reminded people about the previous advice for the protection of everyone from COVID to continue to wear masks and avoid crowds (M. D. N. Kerkhove, press release, 2022). Dr. Maria DeJoseph Van Kerkhove is an infectious disease epidemiologist in the Health Emergencies Program at the World Health Organization.

Ultrastructural morphology of Coronavirus. (Public Health Image Library: https://phil.cdc.gov/Details.aspx?pid=23311, 2020)

INDEX

COVID-19 Resource Center 9, 11
COVID-19 tests 198, 209, 212
COVID-19 treatment 91, 93-5, 100, 106, 217, 221
oral 222
COVID-19 vaccines 11, 25, 63, 75-6, 82-3, 167
COVID-19 variants 9, 25, 82
COVID-19 virus 110, 169
COVID-19 virus outbreak 13
COVID-19and adenovirus 73
COVID complications 191
CoVs 7, 31, 117, 135-6, 149, 250
human 139
CPEO (Chronic progressive external ophthalmoplegia) 247
Cri 245
crisis, economic 153, 155
CVS 210-11
cystic 232
cytokines 40-2, 59, 100-4, 106
cytokinesis 150
cytoplasm 81, 246

D

DA 2, 28, 30, 32, 34, 38, 40, 42, 44, 46, 48, 50, 52, 54, 56
damage 48-9
economic 158
days 17, 94, 99, 195, 202-3, 206, 219-20, 223-4, 250
days of symptom onset 212, 217-18
deaths 8, 17, 50, 64, 93, 104, 163, 184, 186, 190, 216-17, 220, 222-4
DeDiego 136, 139, 144-5
defense 39-40, 56, 69, 152
deletions 116, 131, 135, 137, 245
delivery 159
Delta variants 24-5
demand 166, 251-2
dendritic cells 41, 44

dermal 61
epidermal 61
dengue virus pandemic 17
DENV 17
Department of Defense (DoD) 228
depersonalization 185-6
depression 174, 180-1, 186-8, 191
dermis 61
destroy 39, 41, 69-70, 103
development 6, 42-3, 59, 83, 114, 139, 150, 227, 244-5
dexamethasone 91, 95-7, 99, 107
diagnosis 6-7, 10, 217, 221, 250
differences 1, 39, 223-4, 237-8
dip 211
diphtheria 40, 66, 68, 78
diploid number 243-4
Direct activation of endothelial cells 120
director 9, 212, 214
discovery 18, 27, 33, 99
Discovery of virus 18
diseases 6, 10, 12, 14-16, 21-2, 36-7, 62-4, 66, 100, 116, 153, 176, 182, 184, 247-8
cause 67, 70, 258
inherited 232
mitochondrial 247
multifactorial 238-9
new 88, 91
disorders 37, 234, 237-40, 247, 249
complex 239-40
genetic 232
distribution 83, 218, 225, 234, 237, 248
DLLV, replacing 138
DNA 70-1, 73-5, 229, 231-2, 238, 240, 246
strand of 75
DNA sequence 229-32
DNA vaccines 70-1, 73, 150
doctors 10, 22, 91, 182, 188, 243
DoD (Department of Defense) 228
doi 10-12, 85, 106-8, 119-20, 129, 144-5, 254

[Created with **TExtract** / www.Texyz.com]

Printed in the United States
by Baker & Taylor Publisher Services